Advanced Nursing Series

NURSING CARE OF CHILDREN

Also available:
MODELS, THEORIES AND CONCEPTS
RESEARCH AND ITS APPLICATION
NURSING CARE OF ADULTS

Advanced Nursing Series

NURSING CARE
OF CHILDREN

Edited by

JAMES P. SMITH

OBE, BSc (Soc), MSc, DER, SRN, RNT
BTA Certificate, FRCN, FRSH

Editor of the *Journal of Advanced Nursing*
Visiting Professor of Nursing Studies
Bournemouth University

Blackwell
Science

This collection © 1996 by
Blackwell Science Ltd
Editorial Offices:
Osney Mead, Oxford OX2 0EL
25 John Street, London WC1N 2BL
23 Ainslie Place, Edinburgh EH3 6AJ
238 Main Street, Cambridge,
  Massachusetts 02142, USA
54 University Street, Carlton,
  Victoria 3053, Australia

Other Editorial Offices:
Arnette Blackwell SA
1, rue de Lille, 75007 Paris
France

Blackwell Wissenschafts-Verlag GmbH
Kurfürstendamm 57
10707 Berlin, Germany

Feldgasse 13, A-1238 Wien
Austria

First published 1996

Set by DP Photosetting, Aylesbury, Bucks
Printed and bound in Great Britain by
Hartnolls Ltd, Bodmin, Cornwall

DISTRIBUTORS

Marston Book Services Ltd
PO Box 87
Oxford OX2 0DT
(*Orders:* Tel: 01865 791155
        Fax: 01865 791927
        Telex: 837515)

North America
  Blackwell Science, Inc.
  238 Main Street
  Cambridge, MA 02142
  (*Orders:* Tel: 800 215-1000
          617 876 7000
       Fax: 617 492-5263)

Australia
  Blackwell Science Pty Ltd
  54 University Street
  Carlton, Victoria 3053
  (*Orders:* Tel: 03 347-0300
          Fax: 03 349-3016)

A Catalogue record for this book is available from
the British Library

ISBN 0–632–03995–7

Library of Congress
Cataloging in Publication Data
Nursing care of children/edited by James P. Smith.
      p. cm.—(Advanced nursing series)
    Updated papers originally published in the
  Journal of advanced nursing.
    ISBN 0–632–03995–7
    1. Pediatric nursing.   I. Smith, James P.,
  RNT.   II. Journal of advanced
  nursing.   III. Series.
    [DNLM: 1. Pediatric Nursing—collected
  works.   2. Child Health Services—collected
  works.   WY 159 N967 1996]
  RJ245.N84   1996
  610.73′62—dc20
  DNLM/DLC
  for Library of Congress   95-20874
                                                 CIP

Contents

List of Contributors

H. Huijer Abu-Saad, *RN, PhD*
Professor, Department of Nursing Science, University of Limburg, Maastricht, The Netherlands.

K. Louise Barriball, *BA, RGN*
Research Assistant, Department of Nursing Studies, King's College, University of London, England.

Philip Darbyshire, *RNMH, RSCN, DipN, RNT, MN, PhD*
Senior Lecturer in Health and Nursing Studies, Department of Health and Nursing Studies, Glasgow Caledonian University, Glasgow, Scotland.

Doreen M. Deaves, *BA, MPhil, RGN, RHV*
Health Visitor, Gnosall Health Centre, Stafford, England.

Mary-Lou Ellerton, *RN, MN*
Associate Professor, School of Nursing, Dalhousie University, Halifax, Nova Scotia, Canada.

R.J.G. Halfens, *PhD*
Associate Professor, Department of Nursing Science, University of Limburg, Maastricht, The Netherlands.

J.P.H. Hamers, *RN, MSN*
Doctoral Candidate, Department of Nursing Science, University of Limburg, Maastricht, The Netherlands.

Anne Harris, *RN*
Research Associate, Department of Child Health, University of Bristol, Royal Hospital for Sick Children, Bristol, England.

Eric Hassall, *MBCh, FRCP(C)*
Associate Professor, Paediatrics, and Head, Division of Paediatric Gastroenterology, British Columbia's Children's Hospital, Vancouver, British Columbia, Canada.

Christine E. Inman, *BA, RSCN, RCNT*
Head of Nursing Development, School of Health and Social Welfare, Open University, Milton Keynes, England.

Mary D. Jerrett, *RN, MSc, EdD*
Associate Professor, School of Nursing, Queen's University, Kingston, Ontario, Canada.

Gloria Joachim, *RN, MSN*
Associate Professor, School of Nursing, University of British Columbia, Vancouver, British Columbia, Canada.

Y.J. Lochhead, *BA (Hons), MSc, RGN, RM, RHV*
Research & Development Co-ordinator, Cheshire Community Health Care Trust, Nantwich, Cheshire, England.

Kathleen M. May, *DNSc, RN*
Assistant Professor, Health Services Center, University of Arizona, Tucson, Arizona, USA.

Craig Merriam, *BA, MPA*
Director of Distance Education Programming at Henson College, Dalhousie University, Halifax, Nova Scotia, Canada.

Margaret Redshaw, *BA, PhD*
Research Fellow, Neonatal Nurses Project, Department of Child Health, University of Bristol, Royal Hospital for Sick Children, Bristol, England.

J.N.M. Schumacher, *RN, MSN*
Inservice Educator, Spaarne Ziekenhuis, Heemstede, The Netherlands.

James P. Smith, *OBE, BSc (Soc), MSc, DER, SRN, RNT, BTA Certificate, FRCN, FRSH*
Editor, *Journal of Advanced Nursing*, and Visiting Professor of Nursing Studies, Bournemouth University, England.

Katri Vehviläinen-Julkunen, *RN, PhD*
Professor, Department of Nursing Science, University of Kuopio, Finland.

Alison E. While, *BSc, MSc, PhD, RGN, RHV Cert Ed*
Professor of Community Nursing, Department of Nursing Studies, King's College, University of London, England.

Introduction

JAMES P. SMITH

OBE BSc(Soc) MSc DER SRN RNT BTA Certificate FRCN FRSH

Editor, *Journal of Advanced Nursing* and Visiting Professor of Nursing Studies, Bournemouth University, England

International problems and issues

The first two volumes in the Advanced Nursing Series were entitled *Models, Theories and Concepts* and *Research and its Application*. They were published in 1994.

This volume *Nursing Care of Children*, will complement those earlier publications. It is based on a collection of twelve scholarly papers, published in the *Journal of Advanced Nursing* in the past five years. The contributors are nurses and others, who have updated their original papers to provide readers with sound knowledge bases for the nursing care of children. The delivery of knowledge-based nursing practice will undoubtedly enhance the delivery of quality nursing care to children.

The authors come from Canada, England, Finland, The Netherlands, Scotland and the USA. Their chapters are based on scholarly and research activities conducted in their own countries but, not surprisingly, the problems they focus on and the issues they raise are international problems and issues. Furthermore, as their reference lists illustrate, the chapters are supported by international literature sources.

The chapters focus on health education, disease prevention, information-giving, and many aspects of the care of children (and their families) from conception and birth and throughout childhood. Discussion centres around care at home, in the community, and in hospital inpatient, day care and clinic settings. Consideration is given to the needs of healthy children and those who are acutely and chronically sick.

The art and science of nursing

Dr Lisbeth Hockey (1973), when she was director of the nursing research unit at the University of Edinburgh, Scotland, defined nursing science as 'a unique mix of other sciences with the uniqueness lying in the mix' and she argued that 'nursing is the art of applying nursing science'.

The contents of this publication identify, illustrate and demonstrate the scientific elements of nursing science (or knowledge) and their application to the nursing care of children in different health care settings.

The inevitability of the development of the science of nursing 'is written in nursing's long commitment to human health and welfare', as the American nursing scholar Dr M.E. Rogers (1970) has argued. She also points out that the rapid and unprecedented changes in health needs and health care have created a new urgency for the critical need for a body of scientific knowledge specific to nursing.

The contents of *Nursing Care of Children* go some way to making a noteworthy contribution to nursing's body of knowledge and that should help to promote excellent practice. The book should be of particular use to any nursing student who is studying the nursing care of children in depth at pre-registration or post-registration levels. It will also be a valuable resource for all practising children's nurses.

Home care

The opening chapter by Professor Vehviläinen-Julkunen from Finland is based on a study of how public health nurses and mothers evaluate home visits as part of the maternal and welfare services. In many countries, home visits have traditionally played an important part in the maternal and child welfare services, especially during the post-partum period.

These home visits are assuming an increasingly important role as mothers tend, these days, to spend a very short time in hospital after childbirth, sometimes as little as 12 hours.

Mothers appear to prefer more home visits but the author identified a gap in knowledge about home visits. Little is still known about 'the exact meaning of home visits' in modern services. She therefore attempted to elicit information about home visits from public health nurses working in prenatal and child welfare clinics, and their clients. There were some interesting differences of opinion. Most nurses believed that clients had a choice between home visit or clinic visit. But 47 per cent of the clients believed that they had 'no option'.

Seventy-six per cent of clients, but only 55 per cent of nurses, felt that a general examination of the newborn child was important. These and other findings illustrate how important it is to ascertain the views of users of a service in any evaluation.

But both clients and nurses agreed that an important feature of a home visit was that it enabled the nurse to meet fathers. It is interesting to note that the 'convenience factor' of home visits was stressed to a greater extent by the nurses than by mothers.

Immunization

Immunization against certain infectious diseases is an important aspect of the care of young children. It has certainly helped to control the manifestations of diseases which can kill or seriously damage the health of children (and adults).

Ensuring that there is a high uptake of immunization among children, especially those under five years old, is an important responsibility of general practitioners and public health nurses (health visitors). In Chapter 2, Ms Lochhead, a practising health visitor in England, critically reviews the literature related to immunization default. She points out that the effectiveness of immunization was first demonstrated two centuries ago by Dr Edward Jenner in the UK. As a result of his pioneering work, smallpox has now been eradicated.

Undoubtedly, large scale immunization of children has helped to reduce dramatically the incidences of infectious diseases. But it is important to maintain a high immunization uptake as there are still sporadic cases of diphtheria (usually in unimmunized adults). Furthermore, as the author points out, 'there are significant morbidity and mortality rates associated with measles', because the uptake of measles vaccine has been disappointingly low.

A number of barriers to immunization, among parents, are identified. These include a number of myths and concerns about side-effects. There is also a major state of ignorance about the seriousness of infectious diseases. The author calls for 'a team of professionals providing accurate, consistent and contemporaneous advice, targeted particularly at vulnerable groups'.

Ethno-cultural aspects of care

The populations of most countries of the world now have a rich mix of cultural and ethnic groups. But culture and ethnicity can influence the uptake of child health care and the ways in which parents seek help about their children's health problems.

Dr May from the USA focuses on this in Chapter 3. She describes a research study in which she set out to ascertain the perceptions of Arab–American immigrants about the social networks and social support, and their perceptions of seeking help about child health care.

Dr May found that family and relatives were considered to be the major source of social support by the immigrants. Parents seeking health advice about their children even sought long-distance support from family members living in the Middle-East. Some 70 per cent had network members who were exclusively of the same ethnic group. Some parents felt that they were misunderstood when they went for help to a USA health provider.

Information of this kind is crucially important for nurses for, as the author points out, cultural diversity due to an influx of immigrants is a characteristic of urban areas in many countries now.

Hussein Rassool (1995) has also recently stressed that 'this cultural diversity, with a wide variation of lifestyle, health behaviour, religion and language, has profound effects on their perception and recognition of health problems and ill-health constructed within the paradigm of western medicine and health care system'. There is an important message here for children's nurses.

School nursing

In Chapter 4, two nurses from England, Professor While and Ms Barriball, review the development and present functions of school nursing which was established in the UK in 1908. The early work of the school nurse consisted of screening for infectious diseases, treating minor health problems, and assisting the school medical officer.

During World War II, the school nursing service was made a statutory obligation for health authorities. Initially, the service was provided by health visitors but since then the service has been provided increasingly by registered nurses who may or may not have a specialist post-registration qualification.

The authors assess some of the ongoing debates about routine medical checks and screening of schoolchildren. They also focus on the increasing incidence of longstanding illness in children and young people. They point out that more children are now living with chronic disease, disability and handicap because improved medical management has increased the survival rates of children suffering from these disorders.

A large proportion of 12–16-year-old children appear to have significant health needs and a large number of accidents occur on school premises. The authors point out that the school health service is one of the most under-researched areas of health care provision. That must surely be a challenge for some aspiring nurse researcher. The authors conclude that there is a need for a well-informed health professional to support school children, a contention they support by citing 'the dismal epidemiological data'.

Health education

Health education today is an important contribution which nurses can make to the care of children. In Chapter 5, Ms Deaves, another health visitor practising in England, assesses the value of health education in the prevention of childhood asthma attacks.

She points out that asthma is one of the most common diseases of childhood: about 10 per cent of children suffer from asthma. And new treatments do not appear to have made an impact on morbidity or mortality rates. She therefore conducted a study to assess the effectiveness of health education for a group of asthmatic children aged 3–16 over a 12 months' period. Both children and parents were involved. The study indicated that parents have a tendency to under-assess the severity of the child's asthma. Yet the self-management of asthma requires a great deal of understanding of the condition as well as supportive information from professionals.

Following health education, the author noted some improvement in the manifestations of night symptoms and restricted activities which may indicate that health education can produce improvement in morbidity. The results in general confirm that asthma is a very variable condition which necessitates an individualized programme of care for each child. Ms Deaves makes a number of recommendations about health education programmes in the management of childhood asthma.

Disease prevention

In Chapter 6, prevention and screening are considered by a nurse (Ms Joachim) and a paediatrician (Dr Hassal) from Canada. They assess familial aspects of inflammatory bowel disease in children.

They start by pointing out that despite a lack of knowledge about the cause of inflammatory bowel disease there is an increased prevalence among relatives of patients who suffer from the condition. Their study identified the prevalence of inflammatory bowel disease in family members of affected children. Some 28 per cent of the children had relatives who had the disease. Some of the children had more than one family member suffering from the condition; more frequently the condition was found on the mother's side of the family.

The value of obtaining this kind of information is clear. It would facilitate the development of appropriate preventive and family planning measures and screening for high-risk individuals and families. Early intervention might prevent some of the costly long-range complications for the individual patient and family.

Readers might also conclude therefore that more knowledge about any familial condition would help to improve the quality of care and the quality of life of affected individuals and their families. But I should stress that any condition that is screened for should be capable of amelioration by treatment, a point made tellingly by Dr Godfrey Fowler (1995) of the Radcliffe Infirmary, Oxford, England. He points out that screening is only the beginning. Appropriate counselling, treatment and follow-up are necessary concomitants.

Chronic illness

Dr Jerrett from Canada, in Chapter 7, in her discussion of parents' experiences of learning about the care of a chronically sick child, indicates that the primary source of care for these children is the family. The parents have to manage the child's illness on a daily basis. Her chapter is based on the results of research which investigated the ways in which parents of children with chronic illness (juvenile arthritis) experience their child's illness.

The process the parents go through as they come to terms with managing the child's condition is interpreted as a source of learning. She suggests that there are two ways of thinking about the child's illness: 'First, there is the actual disease of pathology to reckon with and second, there is the perspective of how the disease and treatment affect the parents' role and family life'.

Both fathers and mothers were interviewed and the author identifies the advantages. Two accounts were obtained. Dr Jerrett suggests that a more reliable picture probably emerges from the two accounts as issues in one interview are confirmed or acknowledged in the other. One version might also supplement information not given in the other.

The findings suggest that the parents' initial reactions were confusion and emotional turmoil. They felt unable to cope and had feelings of anger. Emotional responses were, the author indicates, an important part of coming to terms with the situation, leading eventually to an acceptance that they would have to do things differently.

Parents believed that they had personal expertise based on their caring experiences but, also, their relationships with health professionals were far from ideal. The author concludes, rightly, that 'nurses must open the way for improved relationships ... a model that means shared understanding and views the parents as partners involved in shaping their own role as caregivers'.

Day care

For sound psychological and economic reasons, there has been an expansion of day care health services. Provision of day care services means that a child can arrive at a day hospital or unit in the morning, be provided with treatment or surgery, and return home the same day. So hospitalization is avoided. But, as Ms Ellerton and Mr Meriam from Canada point out in Chapter 8, responsibility for preparing children for day care rests largely with the parents.

This chapter describes the evaluation of a programme to prepare children and their parents for day surgery. A nurse met with the parents and reviewed the management of the common side-effects of anaesthesia and surgery. The programme appears to have helped to alleviate the actual levels of stress and anxiety experienced by parents and children. The parents identified the nurse as one of their primary sources of information and were highly satisfied by the information received from nurses.

In Chapter 9, Ms Inman from England focuses on the child in an oncology clinic. Here is an interesting analysis of the child's view and the parents' opinion of the effect of medical encounters at these clinics.

The study shows that a child's apprehension about clinic visits is reduced when staff give the child personal attention, adequate explanations and handle the child sensitively. Children tended to react adversely to excessive gaze by doctors.

Pain relief

Relief of pain and ensuring that children remain pain free are key concerns of nurses. In Chapter 10 Ms Hamers and colleagues from The Netherlands consider the factors influencing nurses' pain assessments and interventions in the care of children.

They note that in clinical practice nurses appear to make different judgements regarding the assessment of pain and the implementation of pain relief. Their chapter reports on two studies in which attempts were made to find out information about the factors which influence nurses' decisions about pain.

The research questions posed were: on the basis of what information do nurses assess acute pain in children and what information do they consider when choosing pain-relieving interventions? The factors found to influence nurses' decisions were: the medical diagnosis, the child's expressions, age and parents, and the knowledge, experience, attitude and workload of the nurse. The nurses' negative views on non-analgesics were striking. It is possible that children receive insufficient analgesics or that analgesics are administered too late to relieve pain appropriately.

Evolving role of the nurse and parents

In Chapter 11, Ms Harris and Dr Redshaw from England discuss the changing role of the neonatal nurse. Over time, all nurses' roles change. Sometimes the discussion about these changed roles centres on the 'expanded' role of the nurse; perhaps a more appropriate way of describing these changes would be to talk about the 'evolving' role of the nurse.

The authors note that as the boundaries of nursing in neonatal care and the interface between nursing and medical practices are changing, inevitably the neonatal nurse's role expands, but this is not universally accepted. The role of the neonatal nurse is a particularly interesting one to study because there have been rapid advances in the knowledge and expertise needed for the increasing numbers of small, sick, newborn babies. And furthermore, the authors point out, the development of the neonatal nurse's role has taken place in a number of countries in response to medical staffing crises.

The study reported in their chapter is part of a large scale study of neonatal units in England. The authors have identified common and technical tasks expected of a neonatal nurse. In some instances, the nurses were involved in invasive procedures. To many of the neonatal nurses, the changing role, in their view, should include training, education and research, and family-centred care. But the authors raise ethical and legal questions about the use of unqualified staff in neonatal units.

This chapter should provide food for thought in discussions about the expanding and developing roles of nurses in the care of children during a time of rapid knowledge creation, medical development and technological innovation in health care.

Finally, in Chapter 12, Dr Darbyshire from Scotland traces the historical development of parental involvement in the care of their children. Historically little or no attempt was made to understand what living in hospitals was like for parents of hospitalized children – or what it was like for the nurses to have them there. If nurses are to continue to advocate and develop a philosophy of care based on mutuality and partnership with parents, then, as Dr Darbyshire concludes, 'nurses need a deeper understanding of the nature of parents' experiences and how these relate to their own nursing practice'.

Conclusion

After reading this book it will be quite clear that the challenges facing nurses who care for children are many and complex. All nurses have to learn to live with constant change in health care organizations, and changes in their own roles. They have to ensure that their roles are cost-effective, adequate and appropriate for the care of children and their families. That requires nurses who are knowledgeable and inquisitive practitioners. It is also important that children's nurses recognize their role as interdependent practitioners with others in the health care team; not only with other professional workers but also with the parents who give so much care to their children during that crucially important time of their lives.

The care that nurses provide for children should always ensure that children themselves give informed consent for any care and treatment that they require. Sick children in particular, and all children in general, need a powerful advocate to ensure that their views are considered at all times. That important point was stressed so well by a paediatric staff nurse, Edward

Purssell (1995), in the *Journal of Advanced Nursing*. 'We need to learn to respect children just as we do adults, both in regard to medical care and generally,' he pleaded. That entails considering children 'as complete entities rather than simply immature adults'.

He concludes: 'Part of this process of learning to value children is to value their views and opinions, even though it is difficult to think of values that are more fundamental than those embodied in the principle of informed medical consent by children'.

References

Fowler, G. (1995) Instant Screening (letters to the editor). *The Times*, 18 March, 19.

Hockey, L. (1973) Nursing Research as a Basis for Nursing Science (unpublished paper). University of Edinburgh, Edinburgh.

Purssell, E. (1995) Listening to children: medical treatment and consent (guest editorial). *Journal of Advanced Nursing*, **21**, 623–4.

Rassool, G.H. (1995) The health status and health care of ethnocultural minorities in the UK: an agenda for action (guest editorial). *Journal of Advanced Nursing*, **21**, 199–221.

Rogers, M.E. (1970) *An Introduction to the Theoretical Basis of Nursing*. Davis, New York.

Chapter 1
The function of home visits in maternal and child welfare as evaluated by service providers and users

KATRI VEHVILÄINEN-JULKUNEN, *RN, PhD*
Professor, Department of Nursing Science, University of Kuopio, Finland

This study looks at how public health nurses and clients of maternal and child welfare clinics evaluate the function and meaning of home visits. Another concern is with the options available to the service user. The data were collected during November and December 1992 from a total of 203 health centres across Finland; responses were obtained from 263 public health nurses and 323 clients. The results are presented in the form of frequencies, percentages and cross tabulations. According to the results, the clients felt that the most important function of home visits was to have a competent professional examination of the newborn. They also attached much importance to the information function, i.e. learning about the growth and care of small children. The public health nurses, on the other hand, felt that the most important function of home visits was to support and encourage parents and to ensure the continuity of care. The advantages of meeting in the client's home environment were equally stressed by both sides. By contrast, clients and public health nurses had very different views on the options available to the client. Almost all nurses said that the client can freely choose between home visits and visiting the clinic; however, only about half the clients felt they could choose the service they best preferred.

Introduction: purpose of the study

Home visits have traditionally been an important part of maternal and child welfare clinic services in Finland. Nursing care in the postpartum period has been considered to be critical in helping mothers and families to cope with a new life situation. As recently as the 1940s and 1950s, home visits were in fact virtually the only way for public health nurses and midwives to meet their clients. They are still an important part of the job; according to a recent study by Kemppainen & Liimatainen (1991), around 10% of all contacts in Finnish prenatal and child welfare clinics are through home visits.

The recommendation is that at least one home visit should be made soon after childbirth, and another visit made at a later date. The latest guidelines for staff working at child welfare clinics (Lastenneuvolaopas 1990) say that home visits provide an important means of family-orientation as well as social proximity. Today, as mothers are staying for shorter periods of time in hospital after childbirth and as outpatient childbirths (mothers staying in hospital for only about 12 hours after childbirth) are gaining in popularity, home visits are also assuming an increasingly important role in health care.

This chapter describes the results of a questionnaire study which measured the attitudes of public health nurses and clients of prenatal and child welfare clinics towards home visits. Home visit refers here to the first visit by a public health nurse to the family; this visit is made after the mother and baby have been discharged from hospital or once the child has been registered as a client of the child welfare clinic, before the age of 2 weeks.

Literature review

Earlier studies on the services provided by prenatal and child welfare clinics have been concerned with expectations attached to the job, its contents and decision-making, relations of interaction, and the impacts of various experiments (Lauri & Hietaranta 1990; Lauri 1991; Rautava *et al.* 1991; Chalmers 1992; Vehviläinen-Julkunen 1992; Vakkilainen 1992; Kaila & Lauri 1992; Vehviläinen-Julkunen 1993; Kendall 1993). The role and function of home visits, on the other hand, has so far received only marginal attention (Hall 1980; Petrowski 1981; Morgan & Barden 1985; Pender 1987; Field & Renfrew (Houston) 1991; Pearson 1991).

Therefore we still know very little about the views of either clients or public health nurses on home visits and what they mean to them (Karjalainen 1992; Varjoranta 1992; Kuronen 1993). The most recent studies suggest that patterns of work at prenatal and child welfare clinics are still fairly mechanical, which means that clients have very little say in determining the nature and frequency of contacts or in the choice of home visits or visits to the clinic (Kristjanson & Chalmers 1991; Field & Renfrew (Houston) 1991; Rautava *et al.* 1991; Lauri 1994; Kuronen 1993).

The research evidence indicates that clients have a definite preference for home visits because they feel insecure with their newborn and because the public health nurse can provide guidance to the whole family in the home environment. One of the studies supporting this view is the work by Lauri & Hietaranta (1990), who were concerned with home visit guidance to families with their first child. Most families found that the guidance they received during home visits was more directly relevant to their needs than the help and guidance they received during visits to the clinic (Hall 1980; Petrowski 1981).

The public health nurses concentrated most on the welfare of the mother and the newborn; least attention was given to health habits. In addition, the clients felt it was important that the whole family was taken into account and that discussions with the public health nurse took place on equal terms in a calm and relaxed manner (Lauri 1991, Vehviläinen-Julkunen 1995).

On the other hand, public health nurses have complained that they do not always have enough time to make home visits (Viljanen & Lauri 1990; Field & Renfrew (Houston) 1991; Kristjanson & Chalmers 1991). According to the results of the observation and interview study by Kuronen (1993), public health nurses consider home visits as genuine situations and as useful opportunities to meet the whole family. However, it seems that the service providers tend to look at these situations from their own point of view rather than considering the benefits to the client.

The interview study by Karjalainen (1992) on home visits by public health nurses from maternal and child welfare clinics uncovered the meanings that families attach to home visits; they thought it was important to have a professional nurse examine their baby, to receive feedback on how they had managed, to receive support and encouragement in child care, and to be able to stay at home in their own, safe environment. In short, clients of maternal and child welfare clinics would prefer public health nurses to visit them at home more frequently. On the other hand, we still know very little about the true options for clients or about the exact meaning of home visits in the modern system of maternal care and child welfare in Finland.

This study is part of a major research project that is interested in the contents and meanings of home visits as a part of nursing in maternal and child health care. The purpose of the study was to find out what sort of options are available to clients and to explore the meanings and functions of home visits from the viewpoint of both clients and public health nurses. The following two questions were addressed:

(1) How do public health nurses and clients describe the options they have with regard to home visits?
(2) How do public health nurses and clients describe the functions and meanings of home visits?

Materials and methods

The information was collected by a postal questionnaire during November and December 1992. The population consisted of all public health nurses working in Finland's prenatal and child welfare clinics. Permission to conduct the study was obtained from top officials in the health centres, municipal boards of health and in some towns from ethical committees (for the client material). At the first stage a letter was mailed to 223 nursing administrators at community health centres, requesting them to send in lists of all public health nurses engaged in prenatal care and child welfare services. In addition, the nursing administrators were requested to specify the public health nurse's scope of responsibilities, that is whether she specialized in prenatal care, child welfare services or comprehensive nursing.

A total of 203 health centres granted permission to carry out the study. The health centres that refused to take part gave the following reasons: they were involved in some other research and development project; they were in the middle of some other major reorganization; the public health nurses were unwilling to take part; or the public health nurses did not make home visits. A systematic random sample of 100 public health nurses was drawn from each of the three categories (prenatal care, child welfare, and comprehensive nursing, the total being 2000 public health nurses), giving a total of 300 public health nurses. Of these, 270 (90%) completed and returned the questionnaire. Questionnaires containing incomplete data were rejected; thus the final response rate was 89% ($n = 263$).

Data

The client data were collected by drawing another systematic random sample of 300 public health nurses. These nurses were requested to mail questionnaires to their last (one or two) home visit clients. Twenty client questionnaires were returned because the nurses had discontinued home visits because of the lack of financial resources in the health centre. The chapter describes the results obtained from 323 clients (response rate 78%).

The questionnaires included both structured and open-ended questions, and they were designed on the basis of existing theoretical knowledge and earlier work in this field (e.g. Lauri 1991; Karjalainen 1992; Varjoranta 1992; Vehviläinen-Julkunen 1992, 1993). The questionnaires for clients and public health nurses were more or less identical, because the purpose was to look at the same phenomena from both clients' and public health nurses' perspective. They were tested in advance with 12 health centre clients and 12 public health nurses; some minor changes were made on this basis. To improve the validity of the indices, expert assessments were also used. The internal consistency of the indices was measured for certain items by Cronbach alpha (Polit & Hungler 1991).

The analysis was carried out using the SPSS/PC + program. The results are presented in the form of descriptive frequencies and percentage distributions. Cross tabulation was used to describe the associations between the public health nurses' work methods and the meaning of home visits. Group differences were tested with the chi-squared test.

Results

Description of the material

All the public health nurses ($n=263$) who took part were women. The oldest respondents were 60 years of age and the youngest 23; their mean age was 44 years. Average career length in prenatal clinics was 9 years (range 0–34 years) and in child welfare clinics 10 years (range 0–35 years). Almost half of them (49%, $n=129$) worked in rural areas, 40% ($n=105$) in urban areas and the remaining 11% ($n=29$) in both urban and rural areas. The majority or 70% ($n=184$) of the respondents were registered public health nurses; 16% ($n=42$) were midwives and 14% ($n=37$) had a combined public health nurse/midwife degree.

The age of the clients varied between 18 and 46 years (mean age 29 years). The vast majority of the clients 91% ($n=295$) lived in a nuclear family, 3% ($n=10$) in an extended family, 1% ($n=3$) in a sole-provider family, and 5% ($n=15$) in a reconstructed family with a stepfather. One-third or 30% ($n=98$) of the clients lived in sparsely populated rural areas, 43% ($n=139$) in population centres and 27% ($n=86$) in urban areas.

Choices related to home visits

Over half of the clients (53%, $n=171$) said that they were given a choice between home visits and visiting the clinic; 47% ($n=152$) said they had no option. By contrast, almost all (90%) of the public health nurses said that the clients have a choice. Over three-quarters (79%, $n=256$) of the clients had themselves contacted the clinic after childbirth and 74% ($n=240$) had arranged for a home visit with the public health nurse in advance. About half (55%, $n=145$) of the public health nurses who made home visits for maternal and child welfare services said they agreed with their clients about home visits in advance. Almost all clients (87%, $n=282$) felt that the time allotted to one home visit was just about right.

Almost all clients (96%, $n=311$) felt that home visits in both services were still necessary; only 4% ($n=12$) were of the opinion that the home visit service could be discontinued if clinic services have to be cut. Less than half (43%, $n=140$) of the clients wanted home visits to continue to preschool age. Similarly, 40% ($n=105$) of the 263 public health nurses were of the opinion that home visits to infants and children of preschool age should be increased. However, over half (54%, $n=142$) felt that the current frequency of home visits was sufficient; 6% of the respondents ($n=16$) did not answer the question.

Meanings of home visits to clients and public health nurses

Three-quarters of the clients (76%, $n=247$) and over half of the public health nurses (55%, $n=145$) said they felt the general examination of the newborn child was very important. About one-third (31%, $n=82$) of the public health nurses thought that weighing the child was of little importance, while among clients 81% ($n=262$) regarded this as very important or important (Table 1.1). The majority (82%, $n=215$) of the public health nurses felt that support and encouragement in child care was a very important function. Only one-quarter of the clients (25%, $n=81$) regarded this as equally important as the nurses.

Public health nurses also attached much importance to the function of instilling a sense of security in the family (71%, $n=187$) and to creating and sustaining cooperation (62%, $n=163$). About half of the clients (48%, $n=156$) emphasized the importance of creating cooperation. Among clients, only one-third (32%, $n=103$) regarded the sense of security as a very important factor (Table 1.2).

Both the public health nurses and the clients agreed that the environment played an important role in home visits (Table 1.3). The nurses considered it very important that the family can remain in its own environment (41%, $n=107$), that the family can be at ease and relaxed (43%, $n=113$), that they also meet the child's father (40%, $n=106$) and that the mother does not need to go to the trouble of visiting the clinic (38%, $n=100$). According to the clients, the most important environmental factors were related to meeting the father (34%, $n=110$) and to the fact that the mother can stay at home (33%, $n=107$).

By contrast, neither the clients nor the public health nurses thought that the factor of peace and quiet was a major consideration in the function of home visits. There were no statistical differences between the views of the public health nurses specializing in child welfare, prenatal care and comprehensive nursing on the importance of home visits.

Discussion

In this chapter I have discussed the meanings attached by providers and users to the home visit services of maternal and child welfare clinics and looked at the opportunities of clients to choose the service they best prefer. While almost all public health nurses said that clients are free to choose between home visits and visiting the clinic, only about half of the clients said they were given a choice. This result is consistent with the findings of earlier studies that refer to the partly normative nature of clinic work (Field & Renfrew (Houston) 1991; Kristjanson & Chalmers 1991; Rautava *et al.* 1991; Kur-

Table 1.1 The meanings of home visits connected to a professional nurse's general examination as seen by public health nurses (PHN) (*n* = 263) and clients (C) (*n* = 323).

	Very important				Important				Do not know				Little importance				Very little importance				Total			
	PHN		C		PHN		C		PHN		C		PHN		C		PHN		C		PHN		C	
	n	%	*n*	%	*n*	%	*n*	%	*n*	%	*n*	%	*n*	%	*n*	%	*n*	%	*n*	%	*n*	%	*n*	%
General examination of the newborn	145	55	247	76	105	40	70	22	4	2	3	1	3	1	0	0	6	2	3	1	263	100	323	100
General examination of the mother	130	49	149	46	100	38	123	38	8	3	15	5	4	2	26	8	21	8	10	3	263	100	323	100
A professional nurse gives feedback on caring for the child	106	40	147	45	124	47	164	51	15	6	0	0	11	4	9	3	7	3	3	1	263	100	323	100
Weighing the child	57	22	84	26	104	40	178	55	8	3	10	3	82	31	45	14	12	4	6	2	263	100	323	100
Examination of the child's skin condition	94	36	98	30	158	60	197	61	3	1	7	2	6	2	19	6	2	1	2	1	263	100	323	100

Table 1.2 The meanings of home visits connected to counselling and information giving as seen by public health nurses (PHN) (n = 263) and clients (C) (n = 323).

	Very important				Important				Do not know				Little importance				Very little importance				Total			
	PHN		C		PHN		C		PHN		C		PHN		C		PHN		C		PHN		C	
	n	%	n	%	n	%	n	%	n	%	n	%	n	%	n	%	n	%	n	%	n	%	n	%
Support and encouragement in child care	215	82	81	25	43	16	174	54	2	1	25	8	3	1	33	10	0	0	10	3	263	100	323	100
Information sharing	91	35	132	41	144	55	183	57	8	3	0	0	13	4	4	1	7	3	4	1	263	100	323	100
Instilling sense of security in the family	187	71	103	32	72	27	165	51	2	1	23	7	2	1	26	8	0	0	6	2	263	100	323	100
Creating/sustaining cooperation	163	62	156	48	87	33	135	42	7	3	10	3	6	2	15	5	0	0	7	2	263	100	323	100

Table 1.3 The meanings of home visits connected to the environment as seen by public health nurses (PHN) (*n* = 263) and clients (C) (*n* = 323).

	Very important				Important				Do not know				Little importance				Very little importance				Total			
	PHN		C		PHN		C		PHN		C		PHN		C		PHN		C		PHN		C	
	n	%	*n*	%	*n*	%	*n*	%	*n*	%	*n*	%	*n*	%	*n*	%	*n*	%	*n*	%	*n*	%	*n*	%
A peaceful environment	50	19	71	22	155	59	185	57	29	11	25	8	22	8	36	11	7	3	6	2	263	100	323	100
Family's own environment	107	41	94	29	129	49	178	55	13	5	23	7	8	3	23	7	6	2	5	2	263	100	323	100
No disturbance	40	15	71	22	142	54	185	57	39	15	29	9	34	13	29	9	8	3	9	3	263	100	323	100
Unofficial feeling	58	22	84	26	129	49	160	50	47	18	48	15	21	8	22	7	8	3	9	3	263	100	323	100
Mother can stay at home	100	38	107	33	126	48	165	51	24	9	16	5	8	3	26	8	5	2	9	3	263	100	323	100
PHN meets the father	106	40	110	34	138	52	129	40	9	4	23	7	5	2	52	16	5	2	9	3	263	100	323	100
Family can be relaxed	113	43	81	25	116	44	155	48	24	9	29	9	5	2	49	15	5	2	9	3	263	100	323	100

onen 1993). On the other hand, both the clients and the public health nurses said that in most cases home visits had been agreed upon in advance, and clients had taken an active part in arranging these visits.

Although it was recognized that the nature of home visits had changed, they were still thought to play an important role in clinic services (cf. Field & Renfrew (Houston) 1991; Karjalainen 1992; Varjoranta 1992). In addition, some of the public health nurses and almost half of the clients were of the opinion that home visit services should also be made available to families with preschool children (Kaila & Lauri 1992).

Public health nurses felt that the most important function of home visits has to do with supporting and encouraging parents in child care and with the sense of security they can instill in families. Frequent reference was also made to the continuity of care. As far as clients are concerned, the most important function of home visits is related to the examination of the newborn carried out by a professional nurse.

Clients also attached much importance to the information function, that is learning about the growth and care of children. For instance, it was widely considered important that the child is weighed during home visits. These results are largely consistent with those of earlier works on examinations at clinics (Lauri & Hietaranta 1990; Lauri 1991; Vehviläinen-Julkunen 1993). The convenience factor for the mother who can stay at home was stressed to a greater extent by public health nurses than by mothers themselves, although both considered it important. In this regard the results do not conform to the study by Kuronen (1993).

Study limitations

The drop out in the public health nurse sample was 10% and that can be considered to be good for a survey. In addition, 79% of the clients returned the questionnaires. Among those who did not answer, many could have been dissatisfied with the home visiting practice. The questionnaires for the clients were mailed by the public health nurses. Although the public health nurses were asked to send the questionnaires to their last home visit clients, they could have chosen their clients. In addition, the questionnaires were fairly lengthy which may have tired the respondents. Both the clients' questionnaire and public health nurses' questionnaire included similar questions concerning the topics. This gives interesting information on the same phenomena in nursing from different viewpoints.

Even though the results of the study cannot be generalized, they describe the Finnish home visiting nursing practice. The results described in this study are based on the instruments whose indices were developed, in part, on the basis of earlier qualitative analyses within our research project.

Suggestions for further research

In our further studies the aim will be to present more in-depth analyses of the meanings of home visits by looking more closely at the responses to the open-ended questions. The results obtained so far provide useful clues for the evaluation and further development of prenatal and child welfare services.

Further research should devote more attention to examining shared decision-making between clients and public health nurses. If outpatient childbirths continue to increase in Finland in the 1990s, home visits from prenatal clinics will certainly assume increasing importance and indeed form a central part of our health care service. In this situation the timing and content of home visits will require serious nursing research and re-evaluation.

References

Chalmers, K.I. (1992) Working with men: an analysis of health visiting practice in families with young children. *International Journal of Nursing Studies*, **29**, 3–16.

Field, P.A. & Renfrew (Houston), M. (1991) Teaching and support: nursing input in the post-partum period. *International Journal of Nursing Studies*, **28**, 131–44.

Hall, L.A. (1980) Effect of teaching on primiparas' perceptions of their newborn. *Nursing Research*, **29**, 317–22.

Kaila, P. & Lauri, S. (1992) Leikki-ikäisen lapsen hoito-ja kasvatus-neuvonnan kehittäminen. Sosiaali-ja terveyshallituksen raportteja 77, VAPK-kustannus, Helsinki.

Karjalainen, K. (1992) Äitiys-ja lastenneuvolan terveydenhoitajan kotikäynnit perheiden näkökulmasta: ammattihenkilön tarkastuksesta tukeen ja kannustukseen. Tutkielma, Kuopion yliopisto, hoitotieteen laitos.

Kemppainen, M-L. & Liimatainen, E. (1991) Terveydenhoitajan työn sisältö asiakaskontakteissa. Tutkielma. Hoitotieteen ja terveydenhuollon hallinnon laitos, Kuopion yliopisto.

Kendall, S. Do health visitors promote client participation? An analysis of the health visitor–client interaction. *Journal of Clinical Nursing*, **2**, 103–9.

Kristjanson, L.J. & Chalmers, K.I. (1991) Preventive work with families: issues facing public health nurses. *Journal of Advanced Nursing*, **16**, 147–53.

Kuronen, M. (1993) Säännöllistä seurantaa ja ohjausta vanhemmuuteen – tutkimus äitiys-ja lastenneuvolan toiminta-käytännöistä. Lisensiaattitutkimus, Tampereen yliopisto, sosiaa-lipolitiikka ja sosiaalityö, yhteiskuntatieteellinen tiedekunta.

Lastenneuvolaopas (1990) Lääkintöhallitus. Lääkintöhallituksen opassarja nro 7. Valtion painatuskeskus, Helsinki.

Lauri, S. & Hietaranta, E. (1990) Terveydenhoitajan tietoperusta ja päätöksenteko lasten terveydenhoidossa. Turun yliopiston julkaisuja, sarja C. Kirjapaino Pika Oy. Turku.

Lauri, S. (1991) Hoitotyön päätöksenteon ja tietoperustan tutkiminen: erilaisia tutkimuksellisia lähestymistapoja ja tutkimustuloksia vuosilta 1976–1991. Turun yliopiston julkaisuja, sarja C, osa 87.

Lauri, S. (1994) Health promotion in child and family health care: the role of the Finnish public health nurse. *Public Health Nursing*, **11**, 32–7.

Morgan, B.S. & Barden, M.E. (1985) Nurse–patient interaction in the home setting. *Public Health Nursing*, **2**, 159–67.

Pearson, P. (1991) Clients' perceptions: the use of case studies in developing theory. *Journal of Advanced Nursing*, **16**, 521–8.

Pender, N.J. (1987) *Health Promotion in Nursing Practice*. Appleton–Century–Crofts, Norwalk, Connecticut.

Petrowski, D.D. (1981) Effectiveness of prenatal and postnatal instruction in postpartum care. *Journal of Obstetrical and Gynaecological Nursing*, **10**, 386–9.

Polit, D.F. & Hungler, B.P. (1991) *Nursing Research. Principles and Methods*, 4th edn. J.B. Lippincott, Pennsylvania.

Rautava, P., Erkkola, R. & Sillanpää, M. (1991) The outcome and experience of first pregnancy in relation to the mother's childbirth knowledge: The Finnish Family Competence Study. *Journal of Advanced Nursing*, **16**, 1226–32.

Vakkilainen, E-L. (1992) (ed.) Sirkkalehti 3. Perusterveydenhuollon ideointi-, tutkimus-ja uudistamisprojektin (ITU) väliraportti. Valtion painatuskeskus, Helsinki.

Varjoranta, P. (1992) Terveyssisarten kotikäynnit suomalaisessa lastenneuvolatyössä vuosina 1944–1972: syöpäläisten torjunnasta keskosten huoltoon. Tutkielma, Kuopion yliopisto, hoitotieteen laitos.

Vehviläinen-Julkunen, K. (1992) Client–public health nurse relationships in child health care: a grounded theory study. *Journal of Advanced Nursing*, **17**, 896–904.

Vehviläinen-Julkunen, K. (1993) The characteristics of clients and public health nurses in child health services interactions. *Scandinavian Journal of Caring Sciences*, **7**, 11–16.

Vehviläinen-Julkunen, K. (1995) Health promotion in families with newborn children at home: clients' views. *Social Sciences in Health*, **1**, 3–13.

Viljanen, K. & Lauri, S. (1990) Perhekeskeisyys lastenneu-volatyössä. Lääkintöhallituksen julkaisuja 157, Valtion painatuskeskus, Helsinki.

Chapter 2
Failure to immunize children under 5 years: a literature review

Y.J. LOCHHEAD, *BA(Hons), MSc, RGN, RM, RHV*

Research & Development Co-ordinator, Cheshire Community Health Care Trust, Nantwich, Cheshire, England

This chapter aims to provide a critical review of the current literature related to immunization default in children under 5 years of age. The author has used a health belief model as the framework for analysis, examining each area in detail. The principal recommendations for practice are addressed and critically evaluated with a concluding summary of the main points raised and the author's recommendation for practice.

Introduction

Immunization provides immunity from infectious diseases and can be inducted either actively or passively. Passive immunity results from administering preformed antibodies in the form of human immunoglobulin. It has an immediate effect but immunity lasts for only a few weeks. Active immunity results from using 'inactivated' or attenuated live organisms or their products (Department of Health 1988). This stimulates the production of antibodies, the levels of which should remain high for months or years if a full course is given.

The effectiveness of immunization was first demonstrated by Dr Edward Jenner who, in 1796, successfully demonstrated that immunizations, using extract from cowpox ulcers, would provide immunity against smallpox. Smallpox, once a massive killer (in 1629, over 3000 people per million died from the disease in England) was declared 'eradicated' by the World Health Organization in 1980 (Lang-Runtz 1984).

Today, the immunization programme offered to all under fives aims to eradicate the diseases which can kill or seriously damage young children (Table 2.1).

Diphtheria, Tetanus, Polio and Hib (primary course)

In the case of diphtheria, immunization has resulted in the virtual elimination of the disease and the organism from the UK; the few cases which have

Table 2.1 Schedule for routine immunization of children under 5 years (Source: Immunization Against Infectious Disease. DoH 1992.)

Vaccine	Age	
Diptheria/tetanus, pertussis, polio and Hib (primary course)	1st dose:	2 months
	2nd dose:	3 months
	3rd dose:	4 months
Measles/mumps/rubella (MMR)	12–18 months	
Diptheria/tetanus and polio Booster MMR if not previously given }	4–5 years	

In some parts of Scotland, the schedule is started at 2 months, and should be completed by 6 months, with intervals between injections of not less than one month.

occurred in recent years have nearly all been imported (DoH 1992). Approximately 10–15 cases of tetanus occur annually with a 20% mortality rate. The highest risk groups are the elderly, with women at greater risk than men (DoH 1992). Poliomyelitis is equally rare today, following the introduction of an effective vaccine. Since 1955, notifications of paralytic poliomyelitis (in England and Wales) have dropped from nearly 4000 to a total of 35 cases between 1974 and 1978. This included 25 cases during 1976 and 1977, in which infection with wild virus occurred in unimmunized persons, demonstrating the continuing need to maintain high levels of immunization uptake. From 1985–1991, 20 cases were reported. 13 were vaccine associated, 5 were imported; the source of infection could not be found in 3 cases, in none of whom could wild virus be detected (DoH 1992).

'Infections due to *haemophilus influenzae* are an important cause of morbidity and mortality, especially in young children' (DoH 1992). Based on studies carried out in Wales and Oxford, England, the estimated annual incidence of invasive Hib disease is 34 per 100 000 children under 5 years. The disease is rare in babies under 3 months of age, but rises progressively during the first year of life. Thereafter, the incidence gradually declines until, by the age of four years, it is relatively uncommon (DoH 1992).

Hib vaccine was introduced into the child immunization programme on 1 October 1992. It is administered at the same time as the diphtheria, tetanus, polio and pertussis but given as a separate injection in a different limb. Uptake of the Hib vaccine has been relatively successful (Fig. 2.1), which has been demonstrated in a subsequent reduction in morbidity. 'Statutory notifications of haemophilus meningitis to the Office of Population Censuses and Surveys have fallen to an all time low. In the first half of 1994, a provisional total of 10 cases in children under 5 years were notified, compared with 191 in the first half of 1991' (PHLS 1994b).

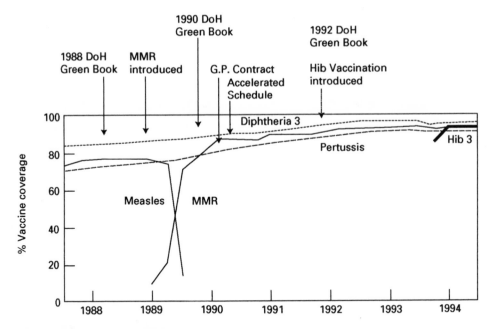

Fig. 2.1 Vaccine Coverage September 1987 to November 1994. Percentage coverage of third dose diptheria and pertussis, single antigen measles, and measles, mumps and rubella (MMR) vaccines (all reporting districts). Data for D3 and pertussis recorded at 18 months until November 1993, thereafter at twelve months. Data for measles recorded at 2 years throughout. *Source:* COVER (cover of vaccination evaluated rapidly scheme) and White *et al.* 'Vaccine Coverage: Recent Trends and Future Prospects'. *BMJ* 1992;304:682–4.

Measles, mumps and rubella (MMR)

Measles immunization has a somewhat chequered history. A safe and effective vaccine has been available since 1968, but vaccine take-up rates were initially disappointing. In October 1988, the combined measles, mumps and rubella vaccine replaced monocomponent measles vaccine with a resultant dramatic increase in protection against measles. This increase is believed to relate to various strategies, including specific campaigns. Despite an overall national and local increase in coverage, there is still wide variation between localities (Li & Taylor 1993). COVER (cover of vaccination evaluated rapidly) data for November 1994 illustrates a district variation of 73–99% (PHLS 1994a). Since the introduction of MMR vaccine, notifications of measles have dropped from 42 125 in 1987 to 9985 in 1991.

There is a significant morbidity and mortality associated with measles. Deaths from measles declined from 1000 in 1940 to an annual average of 13 deaths in the period 1970–1988. More than half the deaths occurred in previously healthy unimmunized children (DoH 1992).

'Before the introduction of MMR vaccine, mumps was the cause of about

1200 hospital admissions each year in England and Wales. In the under 15 age group, it was a common cause of viral meningitis; it can also cause unilateral deafness at any age' (DoH 1992). Immunization has resulted in a progressive reduction in notifications (2924 in 1991) with eventual elimination of the disease anticipated.

Rubella, whilst a mild infectious disease in itself, if contracted in the first 8 to 10 weeks of pregnancy, can result in foetal damage in up to 90% of infants. 'Rubella in children constitutes the most important reservoir of infection from which women become infected' (Dudgeon & Cutting 1991). It was this issue, in part, that the MMR vaccine was intended to address. In the UK the number of cases of congenital rubella is showing a progressive decline, and, with increased emphasis on vaccination, the eventual elimination of congenital rubella should be possible (Dudgeon & Cutting 1992). The situation with regard to whooping cough is somewhat different and will be addressed later.

Thus, substantial progress has been made with regard to addressing these once-dreaded diseases of childhood through the pre-school immunization programme. As stated in the 1992 edition of the *Green Book* by the Joint Committee on Vaccination and Immunization: 'the national targets of 90% for immunization uptake have been attained in England for all vaccines by the second birthday and uptake is showing continuing improvement elsewhere. In the lights of these successes, the uptake targets have been raised to 95% by 1995' (DoH 1992). However, the Joint Committee issues a note of caution stating that it is 'aware of pockets of poor immunization uptake where unprotected children remain at risk, especially in areas of severe social deprivation and among mobile families' (DoH 1992).

The statistics in Fig. 2.1 illustrate how the situation has improved overall and show key landmarks thought to have assisted in bringing about the changes (White *et al.* 1992). However, there is substantial variation between districts, particularly with regard to the MMR vaccination (73–99) (PHLS 1994a). The aim of this chapter is to present a critical review of the literature relating to the failure of the pre-school immunization programme in some areas.

In relation to morbidity, Carter & Jones (1985), in a study of 1492 cases notified in Fife, Scotland, found that 50 required hospital care. Of these, 42% had respiratory complications, 28% had otitis media and 20% had convulsions.

Health belief model

The health belief model, first introduced by Hochbaum in 1958, was constructed to predict preventive health behaviour. Becker *et al.* (1974) illustrate the main elements of perceived susceptibility and severity of the disease, and also, with regard to preventive health behaviour, the perceived benefits and carriers (Figure 2.2). These perceptions are affected by modifying factors, e.g. demographic, sociopsychological and structural variables. The model also emphasizes the importance of 'cues to action' or triggering mechanisms. One can use this model to explore the various factors affecting parents' health behaviour in relation to immunization uptake (Becker *et al.* 1974).

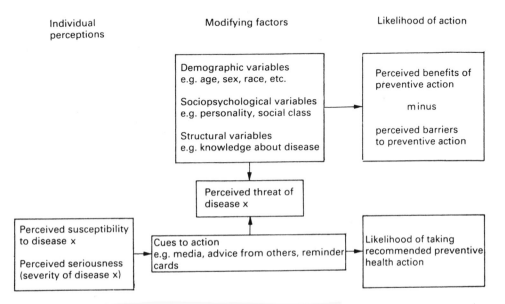

Fig. 2.2   The health belief model as predictor of preventive behaviour.

Perceived susceptibility to the disease

With regard to perceived susceptibility, Rosenblum *et al.* (1981), in a study of 94 randomly selected mothers of children aged 2 to 6 years, concluded that there was no significant difference in perceived vulnerability between compliant and non-compliant mothers with regard to obtaining immunizations for their pre-school children.

Another aspect of perceived susceptibility is the concept of the 'toddler immunization gap'. Chinh *et al.* (1986), in a retrospective survey of immunization levels of children in California in 1985, found a reduction in the uptake of immunizations between the ages of 1 year and pre-school, 'leaving many children unprotected during the years when they are most vulnerable to preventable childhood diseases'. Although this study was carried out in the United States, the conclusions drawn are pertinent to the case in Britain. The authors conclude that the toddler is perceived as 'less vulnerable than the infant', so 'parents may be less concerned about well-child visits to health care providers'.

Dalphinis (1986), in a study of 31 immunization defaulters in Hackney, London, found that 19% of parents believed their child to be less vulnerable because medicine was so advanced that the disease would be easy to control. The same study revealed that 52% of the parents did not receive immunizations themselves, since they had chosen not to immunize their own children.

Perceived seriousness of the disease

With regard to parental belief in the seriousness of the diseases, it has been suggested that parents are unaware, particularly with regard to measles and whooping cough. Dalphinis (1986) found that 51.8% of her sample did not know anything about diphtheria, 42% about tetanus and 38.3% knew nothing about polio: 48.8% did not think whooping cough was a serious disease and 77.4% had the same views regarding measles.

The findings are weakened by the fact that it was a selected sample and, by the author's own admission, the study was too small to generalize the findings to other populations. Reid (1987), in Liverpool, sent questionnaires to a cohort of all 719 child residents born between 1 March and 14 April 1983. He had a response rate of approximately two-thirds. Reid found that the most striking picture to emerge from his study, similar to the Dalphinis (1986) findings, was poor understanding and disbelief by parents, particularly in relation to measles and whooping cough.

Blair *et al.* (1985) found 'serious misconceptions' with regard to measles. In a study of 201 parents attending a child health clinic, only 20% named serious problems caused by measles. This study was weakened by the fact, acknowledged by the author, that 53 of their sample had a child with measles, so had first hand knowledge of the disease. Buchanan & Spencer (1983) express the view that few parents will have had any experience of the diseases due to the initial success of the immunization programme. In this climate, they concluded many parents would get a distorted view of their susceptibility to the diseases.

Perceived benefits

Reid (1987) points out that the vast majority of respondents in his study (93%) were generally in favour of immunizations, but most felt they did not know about the illnesses (87%). However, in the same study, 47% of respondents expressed doubt about the effectiveness of the whooping cough vaccine, 49.1% did not believe that the measles vaccine was usually effective against measles and 15.4% did not know. In addition, Reid received a 46%

unsatisfactory response to the statement: 'whooping cough immunization is rarely dangerous'.

In the study by Blair *et al.* (1985), a substantial majority (63%) of parents thought that immunization was only sometimes or never effective. Elizabeth Moules (1987) suggested that the fact that immunized children may later contract the disease (albeit in attenuated form) could affect parental confidence in the efficacy of immunization.

Perceived barriers

With regard to perceived barriers to immunization, the area of greatest concern for parents appears to be the issue of side-effects of immunizations. In her study, Dalphinis (1986) found that 'more than three quarters of the respondents mentioned side-effects in general and 67% said they were worried about the whooping cough vaccine'.

Concern about possible side-effects of whooping cough immunization is a problem that will not go away. Whooping cough immunization was introduced in 1957, when the average annual notification rate for the disease exceeded 100 000. By 1973, 80% of children were being immunized, with a notification rate that had fallen to around 2400 (DoH 1988). However, by the late 1960s and early 1970s, a series of reports had appeared that linked whooping cough immunization with severe neurological damage. In April 1974, it was made the subject of a television documentary which resulted in the evaporation of professional and public confidence in the safety of the vaccine. Vaccination rates fell to around 30% which was followed by major whooping cough epidemics in 1977/1979 and 1981/1983 (Griffith 1989).

The Department of Health, England, responded to the crises by setting up panels of experts and sponsored research teams, the most well-known of which was the National Childhood Encephalopathy Study (NCES). They studied cases of defined serious neurological disorders arising in children between 2 and 36 months of age, admitted to hospital between mid-1976 and mid-1979. They concluded that 'the estimated attributable risk for those with evidence of subsequent neurological damage was 1 in 310 000 injections' (Griffith 1989).

However, in a recent court case involving a claim for damages in February 1988 (Loveday v. Kenton and The Wellcome Foundation), Lord Justice Stuart-Smith examined the NCES' findings and concluded that 'there were no cases of permanent brain damage or death that can be said to be caused by the vaccine'. He, therefore, would not accept the figure of 1 in 310 000 or 330 000 as the attributable risk of permanent brain damage. 'Any substituted figure would be so small as to be meaningless,' he concluded (Griffith 1989).

Public confidence in the safety of the vaccine has gradually returned with the result that 'in 1991, when uptake had risen to 88% there were only 5207 notifications and the epidemic which had been anticipated failed to materialize (DoH 1992).

Homeopathy

Another possible barrier to acceptable uptake of whooping cough vaccine (it is impossible to be more specific, since there appears to be no statistical evidence) is the belief in the effectiveness of homeopathic whooping cough vaccine. Given the concerns regarding the conventional vaccine, it is understandable that some parents may consider it a viable alternative. However, Dr Angus Nicoll pointed out at an international conference in 1987, that a recent study carried out by a general practitioner (GP) who practised homeopathy, concluded that homeopathic vaccine is not effective. In addition, he suggested that many parents were 'put off when it was pointed out to them that this vaccine was manufactured from the saliva of people suffering from whooping cough' (Cutting 1987).

Poor facilities can act as a further barrier to acceptable immunization uptake. The Dalphinis (1986) study revealed that 16% of the sample felt that the clinic was too far away, 16% disliked the GP (reasons not specified) and 10% disliked the GP's appointment system (total sample: 31 defaulters under 5 years of age). The author accepts that 'a larger sample of respondents would need to be used before conclusions could safely be drawn regarding which aspects need change' (Dalphinis 1986).

Demographic and sociopsychological variables

There appears to be very little research into the relationship between demographic and sociopsychological variables and immunization default, but a few studies have highlighted specific areas of interest. The Dalphinis (1986) study of defaulters in Hackney involved 30 mothers and one divorced father. She found a significant percentage (77%) had more than three children in the family. There were no working mothers in the sample: the author indicated that this was significant since it is often cited as a reason for default. There was a high level of unemployment in the families, but this was commensurate with the general population in the area.

Dalphinis also found that 40% of mothers were aged between 30 and 35, and reasoned: 'these mothers would have been likely to have had their first children during the height of the pertussis vaccine scare'. Reid (1987) concluded that young mothers under 25 years were less likely to immunize. Reid's study was taken from a far larger sample than that of Dalphinis, so could possibly be accepted as having greater significance for the general population.

Rosenblum *et al.* (1981) found 'no difference between complaint and non-complaint subjects in ethnicity, age, income, religion or education'. They go on to cite various studies which indicate the contrary, e.g. Becker *et al.* (1974) who reported that 'poor families demonstrate a lower uptake of immunization than those with higher incomes' and Green (1970) who found that education and income were 'more highly correlated with polio immunization than any other composite of variables'. They also cite an interesting study by Rosenstock *et al.* (1959) which identified two critical factors characterizing individuals who failed to seek polio immunization: personal readiness and situational conditions. They found that many non-compliant subjects showed a lack of persistence and depended heavily on external directional guidance, such as reminders from health professionals.

In a useful comparative study of immunization uptake on a council and adjacent private estate 'in a northern town', Marie Mitchell (1985) found that, in a sample of 30 children on the council estate in 1977, only 46.7% received diphtheria, tetanus and polio immunization compared to 93.8% uptake (sample 32) on the adjacent private estate. The author admits that the samples in both cases were small but the figures were significant at the 5% level. A follow-up study was carried out in 1980 and 1981 which showed a 16.1% increase in overall uptake of diphtheria and tetanus, 18% in polio and 11.4% and 11.6% in whooping cough and measles respectively, but showed similar social class differences from the original study.

More recently, a study by White *et al.* (1992) examined the effects of deprivation, change in the computer system and child population size on uptake of vaccinations. Comparing coverage in 1988 and 1991, they found that 'the more deprived districts achieved lower coverage than the less deprived ones, although the difference in percentage coverage was less in 1991 than 1988'. The size of the child population did not affect uptake but 'districts which changed their computer system between 1988 and 1991, though starting from lower coverage in 1988 than those which did not, achieved similar coverage in 1991'.

Li & Taylor (1993) in examining the factors associated with the uptake of measles, mumps and rubella (MMR) immunization, suggest that it is the relative mobility of families and the temporary nature of their accommodation in deprived areas that may be a key factor, making the families extremely difficult to trace. The authors also identified that children living with one parent and those from larger families were less likely to receive MMR vaccine. The authors go on to discuss the relationship between inner-city status and what they consider to be the key risk factors in achieving high vaccine coverage.

'"Inner city" status has been identified in almost all studies to be an important risk factor associated with childhood immunization uptake.

Although there may be differences in immunization practice between inner city and rural or suburban areas, we believe that the major contribution to lower uptake of immunizations in inner cities is due to the makeup of the population in such disadvantaged areas. For instance, inner city districts tend to have higher proportions of families from minority ethnic groups; in lower social classes, with more children, only one parent, or very young or old mothers; and with more likelihood of being unstable. Such adverse factors seem more likely to directly affect poor immunization uptake than does inner city status.'

Cues to action

Cues to action, both verbal and written, appear to play a vital part in improving the uptake of immunizations. Rosenblum *et al.* (1981) found that the non-compliant subjects in their study 'seemed to need consistent external directional guidance about immunizations'. They state that a typical comment was 'I came back when the public health nurse told me to'.

Marie Mitchell's (1985) study revealed that four out of 13 defaulting clients gave their reasons as 'forgetting the appointment'. Mitchell suggests that this could be interpreted as parental apathy: this, if true, could hide a host of reasons outlined in this paper.

Computer recall systems

Carter & Jones (1985), in discussing the results of their study of the uptake of measles immunization, stated that 'centralized computer recall systems have been known for several years to have a significant effect on immunization uptake rates'. They quote from a study in Glasgow which showed that 'a motivated (general practitioner) practice with such a system can achieve uptake rates of 90%. The weakness in their argument is, however, that they fail to quantify the factors involved in such motivation.

White *et al.* (1992), in their analysis of COVER data, demonstrated that changing the computer system corresponded to appreciably, though not statistically significantly, higher coverage odds. This may be due in part to a real increase in vaccination uptake, but account must be taken of the potential improvement in the quality of the data entered and recorded, as White *et al.* point out.

Health education material

Health education material can provide further cues to action, e.g. leaflets, posters, etc. This aspect does not appear to have been addressed to any great extent in recent studies on immunization. However, Fulginiti (1984) argues strongly that verbal communication alone is insufficient and should be reinforced by 'easy to understand' written documents.

Media influence

Reid's (1987) study in Liverpool established that the media was one of the main sources of negative influence regarding immunization uptake: 164 parents had not consented to whooping cough immunization and 19.9% of these stated that they had received negative influence from television and radio and 25% from newspapers and magazines. This compares with a positive influence rate of 11.6% and 9.8% respectively in this group.

Mitchell's (1985) study of immunization uptake 'in a northern town' revealed that one of the main reasons for default was that the clients had been frightened by television and newspaper reports (7 out of a sample of 32). However, the same question mark hangs over what conclusions can be drawn regarding the general population in view of the sample size, as has been mentioned before.

According to Christina Harding (1985), recent research suggests that 'the media, particularly the press, are commonly used as a source of information about health issues'. The press, Harding argues, must present a topic that is newsworthy and this is best achieved by concentrating on 'events which are negative, abnormal, involve trouble and conflict, and can be personified'. She states that, although these may receive a balanced treatment, it is the concentration on rare events which creates a disproportionate perception of the risks.

In her study, Harding analysed the content of 253 articles about immunization and related diseases from eight British national daily newspapers and eight Sunday newspapers. Her results indicated that there was very little information contained in the articles on immunizations, although it was a frequently occurring topic. She found a 'tendency to describe the negative aspects of immunization without provisos being made about contradictions, etc'.

Advice from others: professional and 'lay' influence

Three questions need to be answered with regard to professional and lay influence on the uptake of immunizations. First, to what extent are they influential? Second, what is the nature of that influence? Third, why do they exhibit that degree of influence?

Reid's (1987) study in Liverpool is once again useful. He split his sample into two groups: 267 who had consented to whooping cough vaccine and 164 who had refused consent. He obtained results on a variety of professional and lay influences, splitting the former into professional groups. Of those who consented to whooping cough vaccine, the greatest positive professional influence came from the health visitor (56.6%) (clinic doctor 49.4% and GP 46.1%). Of those who refused consent, again the health visitor provided the greatest positive influence (39%) (clinic doctor 34.8% and GP 25.6%). This client group received the greatest negative professional influence from GPs (13.4%), health visitors (10.4%) and clinic doctors (9.1%). These figures may reflect, in part, the degree of contact these clients will have had with these professional groups. However, this cannot be entirely the case since the same professional group does not have the greatest positive and negative influence.

These findings by Reid (1987) suggest that lay influence contributes far more to negative than positive influence. Amongst those who consented to whooping cough vaccine, the greatest positive lay influence came from husbands (51.3%) and the greatest negative influence from friends and neighbours. Amongst those who refused consent, the greatest positive lay influence came from the maternal grandmother (20.1%) and the greatest negative influence, interestingly, from husbands (36.6%). Thus, this study indicates the degree of influence exerted by husbands with regard to the uptake of whooping cough vaccine.

Reid (1987) found it 'disappointing' that health professionals were not mentioned more often among the positive influences. However, recent literature suggests that health professionals often have poor knowledge of the contraindications to whooping cough immunizations, and that there also exists a high level of disagreement between professionals (Robertson & Bennett 1987; Nicoll & Ross 1985; Nicoll 1985). For example, in a study involving 40 health visitors and tutors undertaking a seminar on immunizations, Nicoll & Ross (1985) found that 38 were unsure whether antibiotic treatment would render the immunization unsafe or ineffective. If we consider the frequency with which antibiotic therapy is used in under-fives, one can appreciate the implications of such a finding.

Nicoll (1985) argues that a great many mythical contraindications have emerged since the 'scare' regarding whooping cough immunization that occurred in the mid-1970s. According to Nicoll, professional confidence in immunization was severely shaken, providing 'a strong desire for reasons not to immunize'. However, contraindications provided in the DoH guidelines 'provided few legitimate reasons for not immunizing a child' (Nicoll 1985), hence the development of the myths, which were all contraindications. The extent to which the acceptance of these myths as 'reasons against immunization' has affected uptake is not known but would be a useful area for further research.

The *Green Book* first published by the Department of Health in 1988, with subsequent revisions in 1990 and 1992, should have largely addressed this problem, in particular the grey area of contraindications to immunizations.

However, as Kinder *et al.* (1992) state, 'some professionals and parents feel considerable anxiety which precludes a number of eligible children from receiving their immunizations'. The solution they suggest is an immunization advisory clinic 'to provide an immunization referral facility for professionals and parents who (are) unsure about the eligibility of certain children to receive immunization.' This service, the authors argue, 'has contributed considerably to improving the district's immunization rates'.

Recommendations for practice

Rosenblum *et al.* (1981) suggested that:

'... with the diminution in the actual number of cases of communicable diseases, the entire concept of perceived vulnerability needs re-examination. It may be difficult for someone to fear a disease that is not part of that person's environment or past experience. Motivation methods not based on fear or the ability to recall a dreaded disease, need to be investigated as ways of influencing positive health behaviour.'

Perceived seriousness

Jean Orr (1986) addressing the issue of compulsory immunizations, suggested that 'we need to improve awareness of the risks of the diseases' in order to improve immunization rates. Dalphinis (1986) recommended that all the diseases for which immunization is available, are discussed with parents with an emphasis on the severity and long-term effects of the disease. According to Patricia Slack (1982), in a report on a DHSS seminar on immunization, a parent has a right to know what the disease is like and the likelihood of complications as well as the risks from immunizations.

Perceived benefits

Several studies highlighted the problem of poor parental knowledge of the benefits of immunization and lack of confidence in their efficacy. Angus Nicoll (1985) argues that 'it is important to convince the public about the efficacy of immunizations'. One way of achieving this is to 'measure the effectiveness of protection' and to ensure that parents have this information so that they are able to make an informed decision.

Perceived barriers

Inadequate parental knowledge of immunizations and possible side-effects is an issue which must be addressed by professionals. The problem, according to Nicoll (1985), is that professionals are often not in possession of the full facts. His solution is the education of professionals at local level with regard to both the immunizations and the diseases, while addressing the myths currently accepted as reality and dealing with the problems commonly arising in practice. It is important that such training procedures are sustained, so that professionals can be regularly updated.

As a result of interest expressed by other health authorities, Hutchinson *et al.* (nd) devised a model of cascade education where, for instance, trainers from other authorities attend a centre for instruction and receive training materials, so that they may instigate training sessions in their own areas. One problem with this method, acknowledged by the authors, is that 'the message can be diluted or changed' as it moves down the chain from the training centre to the provider in the community. The authors perceive the video, trainers' manual and practical guide to act as a form of quality control.

Practical barriers to adequate immunization uptake revealed in the studies emphasize the need to make clinic facilities more user friendly. Li & Taylor (1993) suggest making immunization sessions more accessible at times when parents find it easier to attend; developing crêche facilities for siblings; and providing opportunistic immunizations when children appear at general practices, health clinics or hospitals for other reasons. Studies by Ross (1992) and Riley *et al.* (1991) demonstrate the effectiveness of such an opportunistic 'catch-up' policy, particularly at school-entry medicals and on admission to hospital.

It has been further suggested that the 'clinic' can be brought to the client. Mitchell (1985) suggests the use of mobile units equipped as immunization clinics situated in areas of under-immunization. To go one step further, several authors have argued cogently for the use of appropriately trained nurses to give immunizations to persistent defaulters (Jefferson *et al.* 1987, MacFarlane 1984). Many still argue that a doctor should be present in case an anaphylactic reaction occurs. However, Jefferson *et al.* (1987) cite a study carried out in 1984 addressing this issue, which indicated that severe anaphylactic reaction occurs very rarely and estimated that 'a nurse giving 100 immunizations a week will encounter such a reaction once in 18 years'.

Li & Taylor (1993) also advocate the provision of a 'domestic immunization service by health visitors or other community staff for families with particular difficulties'.

Demographic and sociopsychological variables

Further research is required into the relationship between immunization default and demographic and sociopsychological variables. The literature studies revealed a possible correlation between social class and poor uptake but (a) it needs to be updated; (b) the samples used by Dalphinis (1986) and Mitchell (1985) are too small to draw any general conclusions; and (c) the samples in both cases were too selective.

The implications for practice from these findings, limited as they are, suggest a need for health professionals to focus on specific groups on a preventive basis, rather than a more generalized response to default.

Ritchie *et al.* (1992) hold the view that community medical officers, in the role of 'immunization facilitators', may be able to lend active support to general practitioners working in practices with lower levels of vaccination uptake. Mitchell (1985) suggests that a visit from the health visitor in the week preceding the immunization appointment could be effective. She argues, however, that this may not be possible given 'caseload pressures'. However, health visitors must address seriously the issue of whether they have a greater impact on the health of the community by offering a universal service or by making it a service based on universal availability while targeting specific areas of need.

It should be said that there is some disagreement amongst authors with regard to the effects of the GP contract introduced in 1990 (Fig. 1). White *et al.* (1992) while acknowledging that the contract may act as an incentive for some, suggest that it 'may exert a perverse influence in areas where general practitioners perceive the likelihood of achieving targets to be slight'.

This view is reinforced by Ritchie *et al.* (1992) who, in citing Wrench *et al.* (1991) state that 'the steady improvement in immunization rates over several years cannot be attributed to recent innovations such as targets in the 1990 contract or the availability of professional guidelines. The view of Ritchie *et al.* is that 'the reasons for the improvement are complex and include much hard work by, and superior educational materials for, all professionals involved – particularly general practitioners, health visitors, community health doctors and local immunization co-ordinators'. White *et al.* (1992) also suggest that improved information systems, the installation of practice computers and stimulation of parental knowledge may have contributed.

Cues to action

Media influence

If the media is 'one of the main sources of negative influence' (Reid 1987), it is vital that health professionals address the fact. Harding (1985) argues that health educators should establish closer links with the media so that a more balanced picture is presented to the public. Slack (1982) advocates 'a policy on relationships with the local press' and argues that this could include up-to-date information on local morbidity and mortality rates for notifiable diseases and immunization levels. Thus, a more balanced picture could be presented to the public, breaking the wall of professional silence which, in the public's mind, may be synonymous with the concealment of the facts.

Advice from others

The whole issue of lay influence with regard to immunization default requires further research, in order that health professionals can target their efforts most appropriately.

The problem of negative professional influence is partially addressed through improved education of professionals, but also by the establishment of a local expert. Such a person could act as a valuable resource, on an on-call basis, available to all professionals involved in immunizations. This would be useful to clarify policy on the grey areas such as prematurity where doubt can often result in inadequate protection. The local expert could also act as a co-ordinator of policies related to immunization, linking these with the ongoing education and updating of professionals.

Professionals also require up-to-date information on the immunization status of their clients to reduce time wastage to a minimum and to target individuals requiring further attention more accurately. Health professionals also need local and national uptake statistics to facilitate analysis and setting of local objectives to improve uptake.

Written cues

Further research is required into the extent to which health education material can influence the uptake of immunizations. It may be helpful for health promotion departments and other health professionals to devise a package of local information related to immunizations, e.g. local immunization statistics, mortality and morbidity, local facilities, and professionals to contact for further information. In addition, health promotion departments working with health professionals and the local media can devise local campaigns which may be especially effective if targeted in areas of increased default.

Legislation for compulsory immunization

Finally, no consideration of immunization default would be complete without addressing the issue of compulsory immunization. Certainly, in the United States for example, it has been extremely successful where voluntary programmes have failed (Lang-Runtz 1984). But the fundamental issue, i.e. the rights of the individual vis-à-vis the rights of the group, must be addressed. Orr (1986) argues that it would be extremely difficult to monitor a programme of compulsory immunization and decide how to deal with 'erring parents'.

Orr (1986) further suggests that 'legislation may further alienate the very parents we wish to help – parents who may already see health and welfare as social control and punitive'. Finally, she argues that it could lead to increased professional control over parents and children at a time when the trend is towards partnership.

Conclusion

Thus, legislation does not seem to be an acceptable or viable alternative. Instead, we must re-examine our present practice in the light of current research and rise to the challenge. Further research is required, particularly into the individual's perception of vulnerability to disease and its associated risks. It is vital to measure the effectiveness of vaccines, to have accurate measures of local uptake, and to ensure that this information is readily available to clients and professionals alike.

Upon these foundations can be built future practice. A team of health professionals providing accurate, consistent and contemporaneous advice, targeted particularly at vulnerable groups – with such an approach, the desired immunization targets could be readily achieved.

References

Becker, M., Drachman, R. & Kirscht, J. (1974) A new approach to explaining sick role behaviour in low income populations. *American Journal of Public Health*, **64**(3), 206.

Blair, S., Shane, N. & McKay, J. (1985) Measles matters, but do parents know? *British Medical Journal*, **290**, 623–4.

Buchanan, N. & Spencer, R. (1983) Immunization non-compliance: time for action. *The Medical Journal of Australia*, 361–2.

Carter, H. & Jones, I.G. (1985) Measles immunization: results of a local programme to increase vaccine uptake. *British Medical Journal*, **290**, 1717–19.

Chinh, T. Le., Jones, M. & Schwaz, P. (1986) Toddler immunization gap. The paediatric forum. *AJDC*, **140**, 615–17.

Cutting, J. (1987) World Health Day: Immunization. *Health Visitor*, **60**, 229.

Dalphinis, J. (1986) Do immunization defaulters know enough about immunization? *Health Visitor*, **59**, 342–4.

DoH (1988) Joint Committee on Vaccination and Immunization: *Immunization Against Infectious Diseases*. HMSO, London.

DoH (1992) Joint Committee on Vaccination and Immunization: *Immunization Against Infectious Diseases*. HMSO, London.

Dudgen, J.A. & Cutting, W. (1991) *Immunization: Principles and Practice*. Chapman and Hall Medical, London.

Fulginiti, V.A. (1984) Parent education for immunizations. *Paediatrics*, **74**, 961–3.

Green, L.W. (1970) Status identity and preventive health behaviour. Cited in Rosenblum *et al.* (1981) *Nursing Research*, **30**(6), 337–42.

Griffith, A.H. (1989) Permanent brain damage and pertussis vaccination: is the end of the saga in sight? *Vaccine*, **7**, 200–201.

Harding, C.M. (1985) Immunization as depicted by the British national press. *Community Medicine*, **7**, 87–98.

Hutchinson, T., Nicoll, A., Polnay, L. & Roden, D. (nd) A training procedure for immunization. Unpublished report. Department of Child Health, University of Nottingham and Community Unit, Nottingham Health Authority.

Jefferson, N., Sleight, G. & MacFarlane, J.A. (1987) Immunization of children by a nurse without a doctor present. *British Medical Journal*, **294**, 423–4.

Kinder, J., Teare, L., Rao, M. Bridgman, G. & Kurian, A. (1992) False contra-indications to childhood immunization. *British Journal of General Practice*, **42**, 160–61.

Lang-Runtz, H. (1984) Immunization: should it be compulsory? *Canadian Medical Association Journal*, **130**, 199–203.

Li, J. & Taylor, B. (1993) Childhood Immunizations and Family Size (Research). *Health Trends*, **25**(1), 16–19.

MacFarlane, J.A. (1984) Whose job is it to give immunization? *Maternal and Child Health*, **9**(10), 302–5.

Mitchell, M. (1985) Disadvantaged children. *Community Outlook*, 27.

Moules, E.M. (1987) Influencing immunization uptake in pre-school children. *Health Visitor*, **60**, 218–20.

Nicoll, A. (1985) Contraindications to whooping cough immunizations: myths or realities? *Lancet*, **1**(8430), 679–81.

Nicoll, A. & Ross, E. (1983) Immunization: reducing the uncertainty. *Health Visitor*, **58**, 285.

Orr, J. (1986) Strong arm of the law. *Nursing Times*, **82**, 34.

PHLS (1994a) Communicable Disease Report COVER (Cover of Vaccination Evaluated Rapidly: 31), **4**, 11.

PHLS (1994b) Public Health Laboratory Service communicable disease report 'Invasive Haemophilus Influenzae Infections: Changing Patterns'. *CDR Weekly*, **4**, 48.

Reid, J.A. (1987) Survey of parents' views on immunization. Unpublished report. Mersey Regional Health Authority, Liverpool.

Riley, D.J., Mughal, M.Z. & Roland, J. (1991) Immunization state of young children admitted to hospital and effectiveness of a ward-based opportunistic immunization policy. *British Medical Journal*, **302**, 31–3.

Ritchie, L.D., Bisset, A.F., Russell, D., Leslie, V. & Thompson, I. (1992) Primary and pre-school immunization in Grampian: progress and the 1990 contract. *British Medical Journal*, **304**, 816–9.

Robertson, C.M. & Bennett, V.J. (1987) Health visitors' views on immunization. *Health Visitor*, **60**, 221–2.

Rosenblum, E.H., Stone, E.J. & Skipper, B.E. (1981) Maternal compliance in immunization of preschoolers as related to health locus of control, health value and perceived vulnerability. *Nursing Research*, **30**(6), 337–42.

Rosenstock, I.M. *et al.* (1959) Why people fail to seek poliomyelitis immunization. *Public Health Reports*, **74**, 98–103.

Ross, G. (1992) Opportunistic 'catch-up' immunization at entrant school medicals: parental attitudes and uptake. *Public Health*, **106**, 143–8.

Slack, P. (1982) A risky equation for health? *Nursing Times*, **78**, 2061–2.

White, J., Gillam, S., Begg, N., Farrington, C. (1992) Vaccine coverage: recent trends and future prospects. *British Medical Journal*, **304**, 682–4.

Wrench, J., McWhirter, M. & Pearson, S. (1991) Childhood Immunization. *British Medical Journal*, **302**, 787–8.

Chapter 3
Middle-Eastern immigrant parents' social networks and help-seeking for child health care

KATHLEEN M. MAY, *DNSc, RN*

Assistant Professor, Health Services Center, University of Arizona, Tucson, Arizona, USA

The purpose of this research was to describe: (a) Arab–American immigrant parents' perceptions of their social networks, including social support; and (b) Arab–American immigrant parents' perceptions of their help-seeking related to child health care. Seventy-three immigrant parents who were Egyptian–American ($n = 17$), Palestinian–American ($n = 44$) and Yemeni–American ($n = 12$) completed the Norbeck Social Support Questionnaire, four Supplementary Social Support Questions, a Support System Map and a Child Health Interview Guide. Family and relatives were perceived as the major source of support and comprised the highest percentage of social network members. Compared with published scores of a normative American sample, the immigrant parents' scores were lower ($P < 0.01$) on all social network and social support variables. There was a moderate negative correlation ($r = 0.47$) between parents' number of years of residence in the USA and percentage of network members living outside the USA ($P < 0.01$) and a weak positive correlation ($r = 0.36$) between number of years in the USA and percentage of network members living close to the parent ($P < 0.01$). Parents' help-seeking for child health care involved use of a variety of resources, with reliance on some long-distance support from family in the Middle-East. This descriptive research provides a basis for further research on patterns of support and help-seeking in immigrant parents.

Introduction

Cultural diversity due to an influx of immigrants is characteristic of urban areas of the United States and other countries. Nurses are increasingly likely to come into contact with clients of diverse cultural orientations who are seeking help for health problems. Research on the social network characteristics of immigrants, the supportiveness of those networks, and how immigrant parents seek help can enhance nursing's knowledge base for working effectively with immigrant families.

Health of Arab–American immigrants

In the nursing and health literature there is little on the health-related characteristics of Middle-Eastern immigrants (Lipson & Meleis 1983) and, specifically within this group, Arab–American immigrants (Meleis 1981). In a study of the health of Middle-Eastern immigrants in the United States, the immigrants identified themselves not only by country of origin but also by cultural, religious, and political affiliation (Meleis *et al.* 1992). An implication for nursing practice is that Middle-Eastern immigrants comprise a heterogeneous population. To give culturally relevant health care, the nurse needs to know not only immigrants' country of origin, but also their perception of their ethnic identity.

There is even less written on Arab–American parents' social networks and help-seeking. Middle-Eastern parents have expressed concern about raising children in the United States (Laffrey *et al.* 1989). In a study of Arab–Americans, they were found to know less than the general American public about AIDS (Kulwicki & Cass 1994). Immigrants from the Middle-East may be isolated from contact with society's major sources of health information. Nurses are in a position to plan ways of disseminating health information to Middle-Eastern immigrant parents, for the benefit of themselves and their children. Health care providers' experiences with Arab–American immigrants (Lipson Meleis 1983) and problematic encounters related to their health care decision-making (Reizian & Meleis 1987) provide an impetus for research in this area.

This research with a Middle-Eastern immigrant community occurred on the West coast of the United States. There is a large Arab–American population in this geographic area, although estimates of the number vary widely. Due to patterns of census data collection, it is likely that the number of Arab–Americans in the USA is underestimated (Nigem 1986). The term Arab–American denotes the three groups studied: Egyptian–American, Palestinian–American and Yemeni–American. The purpose of this research was to describe: (a) Arab–American immigrant parents' perceptions of their social networks, including social support; and (b) their perceptions of their help-seeking practices related to child health care.

Background

Immigrants, culturally and geographically transplanted, experience alteration in availability of their social networks for help with health needs.

Immigration is a life transition for which nurses can provide preventive intervention at vulnerable or critical points (Schumacher & Meleis 1994). In a difficult transition nurses can assist parents and children in coping with adjustment. Immigrant parents' social network characteristics, including support for child health care, have not been explored. The conceptual orientation for this study is derived from the concepts of social network, social support and help-seeking.

Social networks of immigrants

A social network consists of the persons important to an individual, with linkages in the network providing mobilization for various purposes (Whitten & Wolfe 1974). Network characteristics are behavioural and structural (O'Reilly 1988). Behavioural characteristics include emotional support, tangible support and specific support for child health care. Structural characteristics include number of persons in the network, duration and type of relationship, frequency of contact, ethnicity of network members, geographic dispersion (distance of the members from the individual), and recent loss and density of the network. Density is the degree to which network members have a relationship with each other, irrespective of their relationship with the central individual (Hirsch 1980). For example, in a study of widows and students, overall network density was 0.26 (Hirsch 1980) of a possible 1.00.

Research on social networks has addressed various network characteristics. In survey research on Canadian immigrants ($n = > 8000$), homogeneity of ethnicity of the friendship network was associated with low education and with connectedness of the network (Goldlust & Richmond 1974), which is similar to density. Heterogeneity of immigrant friendship network was related to acculturation to Canada.

Migration from one geographical area to another is a major life transition, with complex dynamics varying with stage of migration (Kasl & Berkman 1983). Less than 5 years is considered a brief initial period, 5–10 years a transitional time and over 10 years a long residence (Goldlust & Richmond 1974). In a study of immigrants ($n = 275$) in Toronto for less than 2 years, those who had friends and relatives in Canada depended on social networks for information, although information about available social service programmes was sometimes inaccurate (Nair 1980). College-educated immigrants who spoke English used agencies more than less educated, non English-speaking immigrants. A study of Middle-Eastern immigrants in the United States showed a positive correlation between longer time since immigration and increased social integration in the new country (Meleis *et al.* 1992). In a study of American immigrants in Australia ($n = 60$) social networks were not stable sets of American or Australian members (Bardo &

Bardo 1980). Rather, immigrants usually reflected both premigration and postmigration identities in their networks.

Social support

Although there are various conceptualizations of social support in the literature, the key components of social support in this research are emotional support (affect and affirmation), tangible support (aid) (Kahn 1979) and specific support for child health care. Social support has been associated with positive health behaviours (Zimmerman & Connor 1989), although little is known about social support for parents' health care of children. Social support findings in one culture need to be re-examined for applicability in another culture (Norbeck & Tilden 1988). Examining social network and social support within a cultural context can clarify the meaning of behaviours by persons of the culture (Jacobson 1987).

A qualitative study of 12 Canadian immigrant mothers of young children revealed a gradual change from initial reliance for social support on persons considered kin to inclusion of other members of their culture, then to members of the broader society (Lynam 1985). The women's network use changed as their children's needs changed.

The importance of family and relatives in Middle-Eastern culture has been described in the research literature (Abu Laban 1980; Maloof 1979; Rugh 1984). Little research has been reported regarding social support and Arab–Americans. However, in a study of social support in a non-immigrant Middle-Eastern population, Egyptian cancer patients' scores on perceived social support were higher when compared with scores of a normative American sample (Lindsey *et al.* 1985). The Egyptian sample perceived their largest proportion of support to be from family and relatives, in contrast with a normative American sample, which perceived most support to be from friends (Norbeck *et al.* 1983). The researchers acknowledge the limitations of differences in administration of instruments and lack of matched samples. However, the data provide a basis for comparison with the sample of Arab–American immigrants in this study.

Help-seeking

Help-seeking is the process by which people use or seek to use resources they themselves cannot provide (Gourash 1978). In the research reported here, help-seeking refers to parents' communication or action in order to obtain support, assistance or information about child health from lay or professional resources. People often approach family, friends, neighbours and others in a lay referral system for help before approaching professionals (Friedson 1960; Suchman 1965). In Suchman's research (1965), parochial individuals had more close and exclusive relationships with friends, family and co-ethnics, and delayed seeking professional help. More cosmopolitan individuals had less ethnic identity, more extensive friendship systems and earlier use of professional help.

In a study of Arab–Canadian immigrants, kinship predominated over common community of origin as a source of help (Abu-Laban 1980). In a study of Palestinian–American health practices, immigrant families relied on female relatives who had settled near them as resources in caring for children (Maloof 1979). Reliance on family for help is a pattern typical in the Middle East and provides a variety of benefits, including support (Abu-Laban 1980). In Egypt the strongest affiliation is with the family, which provides a sense of unity and basis for interactions at other levels of society (Rugh 1984). Cultural beliefs and practices which immigrant parents learn in the country of origin, for example in infant feeding (Myntti 1993; Harrison et al. 1993), continue to influence their child care and health practices after immigration. By expressing a nonjudgemental willingness to learn, the nurse can engage the parent in a dialogue toward culturally relevant health care.

Summary

In summary, networks reflect immigrants' sense of identify and may be used as a source of information. Ethnic composition of the network corresponds with density of the network and the immigrant's level of acculturation and level of education. Sources of support for immigrants change over time, and there are limited data on immigrants' perceptions of social support. Help-seeking is related to the composition of the network and involves use of various resources. There has been little research reported on immigrant parents' social networks and help-seeking related to parent health care.

Research questions

The research questions addressed in this research were:

(1) What are Arab–American immigrant parents' perceptions of their social networks, including social support?
(2) What are Arab–American immigrant parents' perceptions of their help-seeking related to child health care?

Research design and statistical analysis

In this cross-sectional study, a descriptive design was used to address the two major research questions. Statistical analysis included descriptive statistics, *t*-tests for independent samples, one-way analysis of variance (ANOVA), chi-square, Pearson product moment correlations and content analysis. The selected level of statistical significance was < 0.05.

Research question 1

Seventy-three Arab–American immigrant parents in a six-county area were contacted through referral from one person to the next, resulting from the researcher's participant observation in the community. After informed consent, all participants were administered questionnaires about their perceptions of their social networks, including social support and support for child health care.

On *t*-tests for independent samples, immigrant parents' scores on the structural network variables of number in the network, duration of relationship, frequency of contact and total network variable (number, duration and frequency) were statistically significantly lower ($P < 0.01$) than scores reported in the literature for a normative adult sample (Norbeck *et al.* 1983). Also on *t*-tests, scores on the behavioural network variables of emotional support, tangible support and total functional variable were statistically significantly lower ($P < 0.01$) than scores for the normative adult sample (Norbeck *et al.* 1983). Network density was analysed using the formula

$$X/[N(N-1)/2]$$

in which $X =$ the number of relationships between members of a network and $N =$ the number of people listed in the network (Hirsch 1979).

Chi-square, *t*-tests and ANOVA of ethnic group (Egyptian–American, Palestinian–American and Yemeni–American) by selected social network and social support variables were done to identify similarities and differences among groups in the sample. To analyse social support variables by gender, *t*-tests for independent samples were used. Pearson product moment correlations and *t*-tests provided analysis of length of time in the USA by proximity or dispersion of network members. Mean scores on specific support for child health care were also obtained.

Research question 2

Parents' help-seeking related to child health care was explored through interview questions. In content analysis (Polit & Hungler 1989) of categorical data, each answer given by a parent was a sampling unit and was sorted according to predetermined categories related to help-seeking, except when responses generated new categories. Chi-square analysis was conducted on help-seeking variables by ethnic group.

Variables/instruments

Measurement of the social network characteristics is described, followed by a description of the measurement of help-seeking.

Social network

The Norbeck Social Support Questionnaire (NSSQ) (Norbeck *et al.* 1981, 1983), based on Kahn's (1979) conceptualization of social support, was used to measure the social network variables of emotional and instrumental social support, number in the network, duration and type of relationship, frequency of contact and recent loss. NSSQ content validity, construct validity, concurrent validity, predictive validity, test–retest reliability, internal consistency reliability, and freedom from social desirability bias have been reported (Norbeck *et al.* 1981, 1983).

In this study, the internal consistency reliabilities of the NSSQ scales were 0.96 for total functional support, 0.97 for emotional support (affect and affirmation), 0.92 for tangible support (aid) and 0.96 for total network. Although most participants were literate in English, the NSSQ was administered as an interview guide rather than as a questionnaire in order to facilitate responses regardless of level of English literacy.

Four researcher-constructed Supplementary Social Support Questions designed in the same format as the NSSQ were used to measure:

(1) Ethnicity of network members.
(2) Geographical dispersion of network members.
(3) Support for child health decision-making.
(4) Support for actual child health care.

Ethnicity of network members was categorized as: same ethnic subgroup as subject; other Arab or Arab–American; or non-Arab or non-Arab–American. For analysis, geographical dispersion was categorized as network members close (within the six-county area) and far (outside the USA).

Social network density was measured by a Support System Map (Hirsch 1980), for which parents drew a diagram of themselves in the centre of all their network members and indicated linkages among the members. Indices of network density can range from 0.00, indicating no linkages among network members, to 1.00, indicating that all network members know each other (Hirsch 1979).

Help-seeking

Help-seeking was explored as part of a researcher-constructed Child Health Interview Guide, which was pilot tested for utility and evaluated by three nurse experts for content validity. The help-seeking questions in the interview addressed: perception of knowledgeable resources, choice of health care provider, sources of referral, and resources used for help.

Sample

The non-probability sample ($n=73$) of 63 mothers and 10 fathers identified themselves as first-generation immigrants of Egyptian, Palestinian and Yemeni ethnicity who had migrated to the USA 1–29 ($\bar{x}=10.6$) years ago from countries they identified as Yemen, Palestine or Israel, and Egypt. Statistically significantly more of the Egyptian–American parents ($n=17$) had been in the USA less than 10 years, as compared with the other immigrant parents ($n=56$), χ^2 (2, $n=73$) = 9.26, $P < 0.01$. Although the researcher had expressed interest in interviewing both parents, more women than men were available. Participants were Egyptian–American mothers ($n=14$) and fathers (n 3), Palestinian–American mothers ($n=40$) and fathers ($n=4$) and Yemeni–American mothers ($n=9$) and fathers ($n=3$).

Parents had from one to six children, with at least one child living at home, ranging in age from 3 weeks to 23 years. The age range of the parents was 21–51 years old. Sixty-nine were married, three widowed and one divorced. Religious affiliation was Muslim ($n=40$), Catholic ($n=10$), Orthodox ($n=10$), Protestant ($n=10$) and none ($n=1$). Education ranged from no formal education to graduate degree.

Procedure

Three years of participant observation and 14 months of administering questionnaires and conducting interviews were spent in a field research context. The purpose of the participant observation was to become acquainted with Arab–American community members, including potential participants, and their child health concerns. In this context the researcher visited community centres, schools, churches, businesses and homes to meet community members and establish trust and communication.

Verbal informed consent was obtained by providing verbal and written explanations in English and a written explanation in Arabic for each potential participant. Native speakers had translated the explanation. Signed informed consent was not solicited, based on the Middle-Eastern tradition of verbal agreement as trustworthy. The questionnaires and semi-structured interviews were completed primarily in homes, at the convenience of the participants. Data collection, averaging 70 minutes in length, was conducted in English by the researchers. Almost all parents were fluent in English and the researcher had studied Arabic, but translator assistance was used in four cases.

Findings

The findings of this research are presented in relation to the two research questions, first addressing social network and secondly addressing help-seeking. Unless otherwise noted, all parents ($n = 73$) answered all questions.

Social network

Size and composition

The mean number of parents' network members was 7.62 (SD 3.7), which can be compared with 12.39 (SD 5.09) for the normative sample (Norbeck *et al.* 1983) and 14.78 (no SD reported) for the Egyptian sample reported in the literature (Lindsey *et al.* 1985). Parents' ($n = 71$) mean duration of relationship with network members was 2–5 years. Regarding type of relationships in the network, the number of family or relatives ($\bar{x} = 4.9$, SD 3.3) in the network was larger than the number of friends ($\bar{x} = 1.2$, SD 1.5).

The parents' ($n = 70$) mean total network score (number in network, duration and frequency of contact) was 69.8 (SD 31.7), which can be compared with the reported normative sample score of 111.93 (SD 44.71) (Norbeck *et al.* 1983). The normative scores used for comparison and statistical analysis were from a female sample because the immigrant sample was predominantly female and because it had been reported that there were no statistically significant differences in normative male and female sample scores (Norbeck *et al.* 1983). All NSSQ scores of the immigrant sample were statistically significantly lower ($P < 0.01$) than those of the normative sample. ANOVA of ethnic group (Egyptian–American, Palestinian–American and Yemeni–American) by NSSQ network variables revealed no differences among the groups.

Loss

Only 27% ($n = 20$) reported having lost an important member of their social network within the past year, reflecting the fact that most had migrated earlier. Many described earlier losses due to migration, including the loss of resources and support for child care.

Ethnicity of network

For 64% ($n = 47$) of the sample, all network members were co-ethnics, i.e. if the subject was Egyptian–American, all network members were Egyptian or Egyptian–American. Most (70%) had network members who were exclusively co-ethnics or other Arab–American.

Geographical dispersion

> Only one parent had no network members in close proximity (the six-county area). The mean percentage of network members in close proximity was 62% (SD 29.4). The mean percentage of network members outside the USA was 26% (SD 28.8). There was a moderate negative correlation ($r = 0.47$) between parents' number of years of residence in the USA and percentage of network members living outside the USA ($P < 0.01$). There was also a weak positive correlation ($r = 0.36$) between number of years in the USA and percentage of network members living close to the parent, i.e. within the six-county area ($P < 0.01$).

Density

> The mean social network density for the sample ($n = 69$) was 0.87. Yemeni–American parents had the densest networks (0.987), indicating that almost all network members knew each other, compared with the Egyptian–American (0.77) and Palestinian–American (0.87) parents.

Social support

> Parents' scores on emotional support, including affect ($\bar{x} = 48.5$, SD 23.9) and affirmation ($\bar{x} = 39.8$, SD $= 20.5$), on tangible support (aid) ($\bar{x} = 34.1$, SD 2.8) and total (emotional and tangible) support ($\bar{x} = 122.4$, SD 7.5) were statistically significantly lower ($P < 0.01$) than scores reported for the normative sample (Norbeck *et al.* 1983). The scores are also lower than those reported for an Egyptian sample (Lindsey *et al.* 1985). Many immigrant parents mentioned that network members would be able to provide more support if they lived closer, but often it was not possible because they lived outside the USA.
>
> The parents indicated family and relatives as the major source of support, followed by spouse or partner. For the normative sample, friends were the major source of support (Norbeck *et al.* 1983). An ANOVA of ethnic group (Egyptian–American, Palestinian–American and Yemeni–American) by NSSQ support variables indicated no statistically significant differences among the groups. Analysis of social support variables by gender revealed no differences in scores of male and female participants, consistent with previous research (Lindsey *et al.* 1985; Norbeck *et al.* 1983).

Social support for child health care

> The two Supplementary Social Support Questions on child health revealed that parents ($n = 69$) perceived more support for making child health deci-

sions than for child health actions, reflecting availability of long-distance consultation in making decisions but less immediate help when action is needed. An ANOVA of ethnic group (Egyptian–American, Palestinian–American and Yemeni–American) by specific social support for child health revealed no differences among the groups.

Help-seeking

Help-seeking questions addressed knowledgeable resources, health care providers, choice of provider, referrals and use of resources. Most frequently parents identified the mother ($n=49$) as the person most knowledgeable about child health care, followed by 'both parents' ($n=14$), the father ($n=7$) or others. Usually the child health care provider was a private physician or health care maintenance organization.

Most parents knew of no Arab–American health care providers, but did not choose health care providers based on ethnicity. Most chose providers based on insurance coverage or financial situation, satisfaction with the quality of care, or referral from someone they knew, usually a relative or Arab–American friend. Other referral sources were professional health care providers, employers, media or a combination of resources. Most parents did not know someone in the Arab–American community who was a knowledgeable resource for health care questions, although many had known such a person in their country of origin.

Parents were almost evenly divided between relying on themselves or relying on others for help with child health concerns. Responses generated the category 'depending on the situation', that is, parents might seek help, depending on the severity of the child health problem. When parents sought help in making a decision about a serious child health problem, the first source of help was a professional health care provider.

Non-serious situations

Most parents handled a non-serious situation themselves or consulted a lay resource. Some parents made telephone calls to family in the Middle East for consultation about child care. Others relied on nearby relatives or a friend because a mother or other relative in the Middle East was less available. It was stated that Middle-Eastern immigrant families are available to each other for help, relying on shared traditional values about family and other relationships. Some parents expressed feeling misunderstood by USA health providers when going to them for help.

Egyptian–American parents and Palestinian–American parents relied on themselves and others almost equally in making decisions about child health. Yemeni–American parents were most likely to depend on themselves for these decisions. Parents who did tend to seek help in making decisions about child health were asked whom they approached first for help. Chi-square of ethnic group by first source of help for a decision on child health revealed that Egyptian–American parents were more likely to seek help from a professional than were Yemeni–American parents χ^2 (2, $n=17$)=6.03, $P < 0.05$, who relied on their lay resources. Palestinian–American parents were equally divided between seeking help from professionals and from lay resources. Analysis of help-seeking by gender revealed no differences in reliance on self or others in child health decision-making, nor in use of lay versus professional resources.

Discussion

This study was conducted to describe Arab–American immigrant parents' social networks and help-seeking. Their social networks and help-seeking reflected a sense of ethnic identity and continuity with their Middle-Eastern roots and a strong affiliation with family and relatives, who were perceived as the major source of support. Parents perceived smaller networks and less support available from their networks as compared with other samples reported in the literature, and attributed loss of support to distance from network members.

Many of the parents' network members were living in the country of origin, less available as a resource for child health care. The negative correlation between number of years in the USA and percentage of network members living outside the USA indicates a potential lack of resources for new immigrants. The difficulty in obtaining tangible support or help is shown in parents' sense of more support for child health decision-making, which can be obtained through long-distance telephone calls, than support when action is needed. The high density scores reflect close networks of interconnected persons, but with much of the network not immediately available due to distance.

Many parents first used lay resources in help-seeking, unless they thought the severity of a child health problem required a professional. Thus, despite the loss of immediate resources through immigration, parents continued to rely on social network members when possible. The Yemeni–Americans' dense networks, tendency to rely on themselves rather than on others for child health decision-making, and tendency to rely on lay resources before professional, reflect less contact with outside resources for child health. Perhaps the Egyptian–American parents' shorter residence in the USA and less dense networks lead to more reliance on professionals for help. Among the three ethnic groups, there were more similarities than differences in social networks and help-seeking, reflecting commonality of Arab–American immigrant experiences.

Recommendations

Limitations in this research include its descriptive nature, from which causality cannot be inferred, and use of a convenience sample, which limits generalizability. Further research should address differences in perceived support and actual support received. A longitudinal study could examine changes in resource use, barriers to care and social support for child health over time. Intervention studies can address which nursing actions are effective in meeting parents' needs for help or information on child health.

Conclusion

The results of this descriptive study have provided a basis for further research on patterns of social network use and help-seeking by immigrant parents. Parents had experienced changes in available relationships and their provision of support. Nurses aware of lay helping networks and help-seeking patterns can identify potential resources for immigrant parents and assist in use of resources for child health needs.

Recognizing the importance of lay resources, especially family and relatives in the networks of Middle-Eastern immigrants, the nurse can acknowledge these relationships and involve them in planning child health care. The nurse's cultural sensitivity can promote a positive relationship with Middle-Eastern immigrant parents for desirable child health outcomes.

Acknowledgements

The author wishes to thank Afaf I. Meleis PhD FAAN RN for her guidance throughout this research. Support for this research was provided in part by a Graduate Opportunity Fellowship, University Patent Fund Awards, and a School of Nursing Century Club Award, University of California, San Francisco.

References

Abu-Laban, C. (1980) *An Olive Branch on the Family Tree: The Arab in Canada.* McLelland and Stewart, Toronto.

Bardo, J.W. & Bardo, D.J. (1980) From settlers to migrants: a symbolic interactionist interpretation of American migration to Australia. In *Studies in Symbolic Interaction*, 3 (Denzin N. ed.), pp. 193–232. JAI Press, Greenwich, Connecticut.

Friedson, E. (1960) Client control and medical practice. *American Journal of Sociology*, **65**, 374–82.

Goldlust, J. & Richmond, A.H. (1974) A multivariate model of immigrant adaptation. *International Migration Review*, **8**, 193–225.

Gourash, N. (1978) Help-seeking: a review of the literature. *American Journal of Community Psychology*, **6**, 413–23.

Harrison, G.G., Zaghloul, S.S., Galal, O.M., & Gabr, A. (1993) Breastfeeding and weaning in a poor urban neighbourhood in Cairo, Egypt: maternal beliefs and perceptions. *Social Science & Medicine*, **36**, 1063–9.

Hirsch, B.J. (1979) Psychological dimensions of social networks: a multimethod analysis. *American Journal of Community Psychology*, **7**, 263–77.

Hirsch, B.J. (1980) Natural support systems and coping with major life changes. *American Journal of Community Psychology*, **8**, 159–72.

Jacobson, D. (1987) The cultural context of social support and support networks. *Medical Anthropology Quarterly*, **1**, 42–61.

Kahn, R.L. (1979) Aging and social support. In *Aging From Birth to Death: Interdisciplinary Perspectives* (ed. M.W. Riley), pp. 77–91. Western Press for the American Association for the Advancement of Science, Boulder, Colorado.

Kasl, S.V. & Berkman, L. (1983) Health consequences of the experience of migration. *Annual Review of Public Health*, **4**, 69–90.

Kulwicki, A. & Cass, P.S. (1994) An assessment of Arab American knowledge, attitudes, and beliefs about AIDS. *Image: Journal of Nursing Scholarship*, **26**, 13–17.

Laffrey, S., Meleis, A.I., Lipson, J.G., Solomon, M. & Omidian, P.A. (1989) Assessing Arab-American health needs. *Social Science and Medicine*, **29**, 877–83.

Lindsey, A.M., Ahmed N. & Dodd, M.J. (1985) Social support: network and quality as perceived by Egyptian cancer patients. *Cancer Nursing*, **8**, 37–82.

Lipson, J.G. & Meleis, A.I. (1983) Cross-cultural medicine: issues in health care of Middle-Eastern patients. *The Western Journal of Medicine*, **139**, 854–61.

Lynam, M.J. (1985) Support networks developed by immigrant women. *Social Science and Medicine*, **21**, 327–33.

Maloof, P.S. (1979) *Medical Beliefs and Practices of Palestinian Americans*. University Microfilms International, Ann Arbor, Michigan.

Meleis, A.I. (1981) The Arab American in the health care system. *American Journal of Nursing*, **81**, 1180–83.

Meleis, A.I., Lipson, J.G., & Paul, S.M. (1992) Ethnicity and health among five Middle Eastern immigrant groups. *Nursing Research*, **41**, 98–103.

Myntti, C. (1993). Social determinants of child health in Yemen . *Social Science & Medicine*, **37**, 223–40.

Nair, M. (1980) New immigrants and social support systems: information seeking patterns in a metropolis. In *Uprooting and Development: Dilemmas of Coping With Modernization* (eds G.V. Coelho & P.I. Ahmed), pp. 401–15. Plenum Press, New York.

Nigem, E.T. (1980) Arab Americans: migration, socioeconomic and demographic characteristics. *International Migration Review*, **20**, 629–45.

Norbeck, J.S., Lindsey, A.M. & Carrieri, V.L. (1981) The development of an instrument to measure social support. *Nursing Research*, **30**, 264–9.

Norbeck, J.S., Lindsey, A.M. & Carrieri, V.L. (1983) Further development of the Norbeck Social Support Questionnaire: normative data and validity testing. *Nursing Research*, **32**, 4–9.

Norbeck, J.S. & Tilden, V.P. (1988) International nursing research in social support: theoretical and methodological issues. *Journal of Advanced Nursing*, **13**, 173–8.

O'Reilly, P. (1988) Methodological issues in social support and social network research. *Social Science and Medicine*, **26**, 863–73.

Polit, D.F. & Hungler, B.P. (1989) *Essentials of Nursing Research*. J.B. Lippincott, Philadelphia.

Reizian, A. & Meleis, A. (1987) Symptoms reported by Arab–American patients on the Cornell Medical Index. *Western Journal of Nursing Research*, **9**, 369–384.

Rugh, A.B. (1984) *Family in Contemporary Egypt*. Syracuse University Press, Syracuse, New York.

Schumacher, K.L., & Meleis, A.I. (1994) Transitions: a central concept in nursing. *Image: Journal of Nursing Scholarship*, **26**, 119–27.

Suchman, E.A. (1965) Social patterns of illness and medical care. *Journal of Health and Human Behavior*, **6**, 2–16.

Whitten, N.E. & Wolfe, H.W. (1974) Network analysis. In *Handbook of Social and Cultural Anthropology* (Honigman, J.J. ed.) Rand McNally, Chicago, pp. 717–746.

Zimmerman, R.S. & Connor, C. (1989) Health promotion in context: the effects of significant others on health behavior change. *Health Education Quarterly*, **16**, 57–75.

Chapter 4
School nursing

ALISON E. WHILE, *BSc, MSc, PhD, RGN, RHV Cert Ed*
Professor of Community Nursing, Department of Nursing Studies, King's College,
University of London, England

and K. LOUISE BARRIBALL, *BA, RGN*
Research Assistant, Department of Nursing Studies, King's College, University of
London, London, England

A review of the literature revealed that the early school nurses were engaged in predominantly screening work and as assistants to the school medical officer. The relatively limited empirical work suggests that they have the potential to make a major contribution to the health of school children; however, their current role appears to vary enormously nationwide in the UK and the issues of competency for the role and integration into the school team need addressing. The consumer/outsider view literature indicated a mismatch between expectations and service provision.

Historical background

The school health service in the UK was established in 1908 in the wake of the realization that 60% of potential army recruits were physically unfit for military service owing to poor vision, carious teeth, heart disease and malnutrition (Interdepartmental Committee on Physical Deterioration 1904). The committee recommended the establishment of a national school health service staffed by full-time professionals rather than an ad-hoc service, which was exemplified by the appointment in 1890 of the first school medical officer by the London School Board (Vine 1991).

The Education (Administrative Provisions) Act of 1907 provided for the appointment of medical officers and school nurses. Section 13 (i) (b) stated that it was the duty of school boards:

'... to provide for the medical inspection of children immediately before, or at the time, or as soon as possible after, their admission to a public elementary school, and on such other occasions as the Board of Education direct'

and also gave

'... the power to make such arrangements as may be sanctioned by the Board of Education for attending to the health and physical condition of the children educated in public elementary schools.'

The work of an early school nurse, as described in detail by Baly (1987), consisted of screening for infectious and contagious diseases as well as treating minor health problems and assisting the school medical officer in his work. However, like many changes brought about by legislation, limited resourcing meant that the ambitions of the service were not fully realized although Henderson (1976) has noted that the young potential army recruits for World War II had relatively good health as compared with the older potential recruits who had been subject to child health services earlier in the century.

Impetus for legislation

World War II provided the impetus for the introduction of much social welfare legislation and included among the post-war Acts of Parliament was the Education Act of 1944 which placed a statutory obligation upon health authorities to provide a school nursing service as part of health provision for all school children, an obligation which has continued through to the present day. The 1977 National Health Service Act stated that:

'It is the Secretary of State's duty:
(a) to provide for the medical and dental inspection at appropriate inter-vals of pupils in attendance at schools maintained by local education authorities and for the medical and dental treatment of such pupils' (para 5 (1) (1)).

In the immediate post-war period health visitors usually provided the service and although in some parts of the UK health visitors continue in the work, trained nurses are increasingly engaged in fulfilling this role. The Court Report (DHSS 1976) recommended a specialist short training to provide school nurses with additional relevant training to supplement their registered general nurse qualification. However, current training has been severely criticized not only for its extent but also its structure (Riches 1980; Staunton 1985). Collis (1985) has made a strong case for educating school nurses. However, she highlighted the difficulties in providing an appropriate course when the role of school nurse varies considerably in different health authorities.

A further confounding factor is lack of information about the ratio of trained to untrained (in terms of supplementary education) nurses employed as school nurses and any evaluative work regarding role performance of trained and untrained school nurses. The recent survey by the Amalgamated

School Nurses' Association (ASNA) (Fletcher & Balding 1992) revealed a 3:1 ratio of trained:untrained school nurses but it was a self-selected group of respondents with the survey suffering a 66% non-response rate. English National Board statistics (Table 4.1) suggest that there has been a reduction in the number of nurses successfully completing the school nurse course since a peak in 1985.

Table 4.1   Numbers successfully completing the school nurse certificate course (Source ENB Statistics).

01.04.78–31.03.79	36
01.04.79–31.03.80	90
01.04.80–31.03.81	209
01.04.81–31.03.82	293
01.04.82–31.03.83	308
01.04.83–31.03.84	306
01.04.84–31.03.85	421
01.04.85–31.03.86	404
01.04.86–31.03.87	358
01.04.87–31.03.88	311
01.04.88–31.03.89	292
01.04.89–31.03.90	234
01.04.90–31.03.91	283
01.04.91–31.04.92	248
01.04.92–31.04.93	164
01.04.93–31.04.94	157

A 1981 survey of school nurses ($n = 282$), however, indicated that there was a strong desire among school nurses for a national training, with 100% claiming they would be prepared to follow such a course even though it might require them to undertake some travelling to the college (HVA School Nurses' Group 1981). The publication of the document on the future of professional practice by the United Kingdom Central Council outlined the basis for national courses which are to be offered at degree level and result in specialist registration status (UKCC 1994). But nurses will have to be sponsored by their employing NHS trusts to undertake these courses, and that might limit the numbers.

Present practice and possibilities

The Court Report (DHSS 1976) was the first enquiry to examine critically the provision of health care for school children since the inception of the National Health Service. Among many other recommendations, this report stressed the need for strengthening the school health service with an improved nursing provision so that the school nurse could function effectively as 'the representative of health in the everyday life of the school'.

Indeed, the report argued that this important contribution is frequently overlooked and undervalued.

While several more recent small-scale studies and personal reviews have explored the work undertaken by school nurses (e.g. Whitmore *et al.* 1982a, 1982b; Staunton 1983; Johnstone 1986), Thurmott's (1976) exploratory survey of the school nursing service in an English county in 1973 remains the most detailed empirical analysis of the work undertaken by school nurses. However, her sample consisted of 58 generic health visitors who undertook school health duties as part of their role and the data was collected by means of questionnaires requiring recall of the previous week's work activities. Since that survey, others have documented the value of school nurses in the field of health surveillance and screening (Whitmore *et al.* 1982a; Whyte 1984; Kennedy 1988; Leff 1989).

There is a continuing debate about the value of regular school medicals for apparently 'healthy' children. In 1976 the Court Report (DHSS 1976) advocated a more selective approach to target those with the greatest health needs. However, the Committee also recommended that universal routine health surveillance should be undertaken by school nurses. Whitmore & Bax (1990) have suggested that up until the middle of the 1980s 90% of district health authorities favoured routine medical examination of 5-year-olds. However, today the need for routine medical examinations for school entrants is under review.

On the basis of a small study of two schools in North Kensington, London, ($n = 52$ children), Richman & Miles (1990) have argued that universal health interviews by the school nurse are more appropriate as children with problems benefit from the extra medical time available to them. Indeed, Kennedy's (1988) audit of school health records of 1033 children in Newtonabbey, Northern Ireland, revealed that routine medicals yield only a few new health problems and that most could have been detected by screening tests performed by the school nurse.

Lucas (1980) also had similar findings. The results of a retrospective study (Smith *et al.* 1989) of school medical records of 100 children born in 1981 also demonstrated that the 5-year school medical was unnecessary, providing strict criteria for the selection for examination by a school doctor were followed. However, Jones & Gordon's (1992) survey found that the majority (78%) of teachers value the school entry medical examination and Jones *et al.* (1989) found a high number of previously undetected problems revealed by pre-school medical examinations in Macclesfield Health Authority.

Routine medical checks

Whitmore & Bax (1990) are strong supporters of routine medical checks of all school entrants drawing upon the evidence of an audit of school health records in 12 primary schools in Paddington, London ($n = 351$ children) and have argued that a selective rather than a universal approach will undermine an effective surveillance of the health needs of children at school. Although they recognize the manpower implications, they are unpersuaded by Hall's (1989a, 1991) recommendation for selectivity. These issues have been vigorously debated in the professional press (Bax & Whitmore 1989; Hall 1989b, 1989c; Law 1989; Squire & Dowell 1989; Potrykus 1990).

However, in spite of this there is little current information (Audit Commission 1994) as to the extent routine medical examinations are still performed for school entrants in the UK, indicating a need for some empirical work. The Audit Commission (1994) also noted that information transfer between the pre-school community health services and the school health service was haphazard, although they anticipated that the introduction of parent-held records would improve information transfer. Further, the limited research reviewing the adequacy of screening procedures is not encouraging. For example, Nietupska & Harding (1982) found the extent of hearing loss among the 30 8-year-old children in their pilot study to be far in excess of that recorded in the school health records when the same children had purportedly had auditory screening between 5 and 6 years of age, although they noted only two-thirds attended the screening session.

While & Bamunoba (1992) also found that screening procedures fell short of the 100% ideal with presumably similar consequences for the children; indeed, approximately 4% never had their hearing tested, their weight or height measured during the first 6 years of compulsory schooling. The audit of the records was undertaken at the end of the children's twelfth year and, interestingly, only 89% of children were recorded as having had a colour vision assessment using Ishihara plates. This is disappointing in view of Smith & Fellner (1985) who demonstrated that commitment to a target can achieve 97.2% uptake of a prophylactic measure.

The contribution of school nurses to screening and surveillance work appears to vary enormously and the variability appears to be based more upon ad-hoc regional policies than on an effective assessment and evaluation of the area's population needs (Harrison & Gretton 1986). Indeed, Harrison & Gretton were impressed by the lack of uniformity revealed by their survey of 128 health authorities.

Tuke (1990) has advocated the reactive model of school health services developed in Northumberland (O'Callaghan & Colver 1987). However, he was cautious in accepting the need for greater uniformity in provision in case current services reflect an unevaluated equilibrium with local health needs. Indeed, he stated that:

> Contact between a school nurse and children in a particular area, on whatever pretext, may have hidden merits.

Similarly, the Audit Commission (1994), while supporting a selective approach in general, acknowledged that it may be appropriate to target certain schools for universal school entrance medical examination where a review of the population and the environment indicates the likelihood of many health needs among the school children.

Screening

There is a considerable wealth of evidence that children develop health problems during their school careers (e.g. Speight *et al.* 1983, McMaster 1984, Stewart-Brown & Haslam 1987). Further, Dickson (1984) had advocated screening for scoliosis in order to detect the disease at an early stage when it is amenable to treatment. Macnab (1987), drawing upon a small survey of 12 general practitioners and three ophthalmologists, has argued for hypertension screening of school children, and Kelsall & Watson (1990) have demonstrated that school nurses are able to include blood pressure measurements in their routine work to identify children possibly in need of treatment. This sample of nurses further identified the monitoring of blood pressure as enhancing their health-promotion role by helping them to reinforce general advice regarding diet and smoking.

However, Hall (1991) is hesitant to recommend universal screening for hypertension at present, drawing upon the North American research of Fixler & Pennock (1983). However, these studies suggest that school nurses can offer an important contribution to the screening of school children, even though much of their work has hitherto been concerned with body measurement and vision testing, including the detection of colour vision defects (Fyfe & Ellerbroek 1984).

While the incidence of infectious diseases has declined, a substantial number of school children have health problems as evidenced by data from the General Household Survey (OPCS 1988) which show increasing incidence of longstanding illness in children and young people of both sexes. Improved medical management has also increased the survival rate of many sick children, so that more children are living with chronic disease, disabilities and handicaps (Bone & Meltzer 1989).

Thus, while there appears to have been some improvement in physical health, as evidenced by increased height (Rona & Chinn 1984), this improvement seems to have occurred with an increased incidence of obesity (Stark *et al.* 1986) and anorexia nervosa (Graham 1986). Indeed, conquered health problems such as severe malnutrition and infectious diseases appear to have been replaced by new ones such as drug and solvent abuse (Diamond *et al.* 1988), alcohol abuse (Plant *et al.* 1985), cigarette smoking (Dobbs & Marsh 1985), teenage pregnancies (Royal College of Obstetricians and

Gynaecologists 1991), sexually transmitted disease (National Children's Bureau 1987) and suicide (Hawton 1982).

In 1992 about 48 000 teenagers in England and Wales had a baby (OPCS 1993), representing approximately 7% of all births. Unfortunately such pregnancies have been found to be associated with poor health outcomes (Konje et al 1992) as well as poor educational and occupational outcomes (Lawson & Rhode 1993).

Further, a very recent questionnaire survey ($n = 23\,928$) of 12–16-year-old school children has suggested that a large proportion have significant health needs (Balding 1992). It can therefore be argued that the need for a well-informed health professional to support school children and their staff is evident from the dismal epidemiological data.

The school attendance of children with disfiguring ailments and those returning after treatment for a life-threatening illness also creates a need for health support within the educational environment if full integration into school life is to be achieved (Street 1981; Larcombe 1991). The Audit Commission (1994) noted that the growing number of children with special needs in mainstream education requires effective health care support in the educational setting and of particular note is the burgeoning incidence of childhood asthma. This had also been noted earlier (Audit Commission 1993). Indeed, the poor educational attainment of children with frequent school absences due to ill health in the National Child Development Study (Essen & Wedge 1982) suggests that greater resource focusing may improve educational outcome.

In addition, the appalling accident statistics (OPCS Monitor 1989) indicate that current strategies have been ineffective in improving this important cause of morbidity and mortality. Particularly worrying is the role of alcohol in the rate of motor vehicle accidents among 15–19-year-old males (Department of Transport 1990) although, interestingly, a significant number of all types of accidents also occur on educational institution premises (Department of Trade and Industry 1989). Indeed, Forthergill & Hashemi (1991) noted that over half the injuries presenting in their accident and emergency department study occurred during free recreational time at school, which 51% of the children claimed was unsupervised.

Training for school nurses

The aim of a health appraisal by the school nurse at any age is to develop a holistic profile of the needs of each individual child of school age (Holt 1990a). While there remains no national policy in the UK for addressing the expanded role of school nurses in health interviews, feedback from several pilot studies and reviews is favourable, not least with children, parents, teachers and nurses themselves (Wade *et al.* 1989; Holt 1990b; Richman & Miles 1990).

However, it must remain of some concern that increasing responsibility for the promotion of health and prevention of ill health and the early detection of problems in the school-aged child is falling on school nurses, many of whom do not hold a specialist qualification nor a definite role description. There remains a gap in the literature about the expected nurse competencies needed to fulfil the expanding role of the school nurse, although the recent UKCC (1994) publication is helpful.

Interestingly the UKCC does not refer to competence in the domain of vaccination and immunisation administration despite school nurses having provided the majority of manpower for the national immunisation of school children in November 1994. Further, such activities are an integral part of the school nurse's role in some parts of the UK (Saffin, 1992). The Audit Commission (1994) also noted that while head teachers identified school nurses as sources of advice and health education, the interviewed school nurses found that suitable training for this role was not always available.

In Latham's (1981) assessment of the pilot scheme for health surveillance in the Nottingham area, she commented that adequate in-service training for school nurses existed to ensure the standard of expertise needed for school nurses to perform their extended role in health appraisal/surveillance safely and effectively, although she did not elaborate upon how competency was assessed. Leff (1989) also pointed out that the school nurse who took part in 14+ health care interviews in Uckfield, West Sussex, had had special training. However, it should not be assumed that all nurses involved in these extended roles have been adequately prepared.

A survey of Californian school nurses ($n = 1227$) revealed that many respondents felt lacking in the very skills which their new role demanded of them, notably physical assessment and screening, including hearing and vision (Brajkovich & Madison 1986). Thus, while there seems to be a lack of UK-based empirical data, evidence from the United States suggests that there is a skill gap which promises to widen to the detriment of the health of the school child.

The existence of a skill gap related to the extended role of school nurses also raises questions of quality assurance of nursing performance and practice in the school setting. While there have been attempts to standardize the evaluation of school nursing practice in the United States (Proctor 1986), this review of the literature failed to produce similar projects in the UK.

Despite areas of concern, Latham (1981) has stated:

... it could be hypothesized that the regular surveillance of children to identify health problems and observe deviation from the normal could be one of the most important contributions made by the nurse to the school health service.

Health care interviews

Two of the main benefits of health care interviews above medical examinations, repeatedly cited in the literature, is the opportunity for children and parents to express their needs and concerns (Holt 1990b; Richman & Miles 1990) and the increased opportunity it affords the school nurse to participate in health education and promotion. The ability of children to raise their own concerns about health issues, provided they are given the opportunity to do so as, for example, in a well-structured health care interview, should not be underestimated.

A case study (Hughes & Gordon 1988) of a group of children aged 4–16 years with St Thomas's (now West Lambeth) Community Health Council in London clearly emphasized the need for professionals to take the concerns of children seriously and to recognize their potential for benefiting from health education input. Wade *et al.* (1989) commented in their review of health care interviews in Brighton Health District that health care interviews with a school nurse revealed more information about emotional problems than routine medicals. Whilst the detection of physical defects is still an important part of the work carried out by the school health service, a move towards health care interviews is, in part, a response to the fact that the service has developed far beyond its original aims (Leff 1989).

In a climate where children are increasingly exposed to health-threatening trends such as stress, drug and alcohol abuse, eating disorders and child abuse, a point of contact with an informative but neutral source in the school setting is seen as increasingly important. Nevertheless, the success of such a provision will clearly be determined by the quality of the staff employed. Wade *et al.* (1989) have emphasized the need for the standardization of criteria for recalling children for a further health review as a means of ensuring satisfactory selection procedures and thereby providing guidelines for role performance.

Carpenter (1985) has argued that not only should the school health service promote physical and emotional health so that school children benefit fully from their education but it should also prepare children for optimum health in adult life. Indeed, Carpenter considered promotion of good health to be one of the school nurse's major responsibilities so that children have the best possible understanding of their bodies and health status, and how they may maintain or even improve their health throughout their life. This conception of the school nurse as a health educator is reflected in a number of papers by practising British school nurses (Holliday *et al.* 1984; Eckersall 1985; Nelson 1989).

Two American studies suggest that the school nurse is able to play an important role in successfully promoting health awareness among school children. One study took the form of an experimental design concerning the development of health knowledge (Feuerstein & Galli 1983) while the other was an evaluation of a five-session education programme (Hufford & Lipnickey 1987). Indeed, the need for more health education has been identified by British teenagers in a survey of 1418 fourth-year secondary-school pupils (Challener 1990).

Similarly, the very limited understanding of AIDS and HIV (White *et al.* 1988) makes it imperative that opportunities for giving information are not lost. However, Challener (1990) cautioned that current health education initiatives are inappropriate and advocated a more acceptable model so that health messages are not discounted by adolescents as irrelevant. Whitmore *et al.* (1982a,b) have noted that most formal health education in schools is undertaken by teachers, although there is increasing evidence that nurses are engaged in such work (Gunatilleke 1992; Jones 1992; Lenderyou 1993). Of particular note is compulsory sex education in all schools unless parents formally request their child is withdrawn from such sessions, by virtue of the Education Act 1993 (HMSO 1993).

National school curriculum

This trend is likely to have been formalized by the pressure placed upon the school timetable by the introduction of the National Curriculum. In view of this, school nurses should perhaps be developing their role as advisers to teachers and as providers of health education resources, both for use by teachers and as displays for children in their schools. Reid & Massey (1986) have made several useful recommendations for improving the effectiveness of school health education, which include a closer co-operation between the teachers and health service staff. However, a close relationship between teachers and school nurses is not evident in the limited survey evidence available (Staunton 1983; Hanson 1987; Jones 1992; Jones & Gordon 1992).

Turner (1986) has described a proactive health education resource service in South Birmingham Health Authority, which provides a possible role model for elsewhere. The competency of school nurses as health educators in 'a formal setting' has not been fully evaluated. However, the perception of parents that school nurses may not be well suited to this work (Fahey & Cutting 1988) cannot be discounted because, unlike teachers, they will be unlikely to have had formal training in teaching methods.

A small study undertaken by Goodeve (1991) in the London area suggests that, while school nurses identified health education as an important part of their work, they experienced considerable difficulties in handling formal teaching sessions, especially those covering sensitive topics such as HIV/

AIDS. Brajkovich & Madison (1986) had a similar finding in their large questionnaire study. The potential of school nurses as facilitators has perhaps yet to be realized.

Plamping *et al.* (1980) have described a successful children's health club, in which peer teaching, or children teaching other children, was facilitated originally by a dental officer. Indeed, the club is highlighted as an exemplar of good practice by the King's Fund (Hughes & Gordon 1988) and exploits the reality that children are more eager to learn about a subject when there is a full acknowledgement of their interests and involvement in the health education process (Moon 1987).

Individual health counselling

The preference for individual health counselling also needs acknowledgement if sensitive health subjects are to be adequately explored with adolescents. Whyte (1984) commented upon the preference among some school children ($n = 50$) for individual rather than group health interviews. The Court Report (DHSS 1976) advocated individual interviews and opportunities for self-referral for all adolescents so that difficulties regarding access to professional help could be minimized. Wade *et al.* (1989) noted that the introduction of health care interviews among secondary school children ($n = 2411$) was well received by staff, children and parents alike. The issue of access to health care is important, since barriers will reduce access to additional health care, the lack of which may interfere with educational attainment.

Brand's (1980) personal review of her own participation in health promotion discussion groups with 14-year-olds in Cambridge Area Health Authority reported that the level of regular smoking and drinking habits already established in this age group, coupled with identified psychological and emotional problems, indicated the need for this adolescent age group to have access to good-quality health promotion. This, then, perhaps points to the need for greater health education at an earlier age before anti-health behavioural patterns are established.

Furthermore, the increasingly sensitive nature of factors influencing the health status of school children indicates that potential benefits could be drawn from regular counselling or contact on a one-to-one basis with a health professional. It could be argued that, within the structure of the school health service, this can best be realized through utilizing the school nurse at health care interviews and additional sessions where appropriate. While the contributions of school nurses to health education are largely outside the classroom and on an informal basis, Bailey (1989) pointed out the significance of this contribution, and the potential of school nurses as health educators, must not be undervalued.

However, the evidence from Johnstone's (1986) analysis of the work content of 23 nurses over a 1-week period indicated that only 5.5% of their time on average was spent on health education and this is despite the results of a questionnaire sent out to school nurses to which 282 responded (HVA School Nurses' Group 1981), in which 90% expressed a desire to be health educators.

Interestingly, 99% of the ASNA survey (Fletcher & Balding 1992) respondents claimed involvement in health education, although the ambiguous nature of the question did not require any quantification of this involvement, so leaving the exact contribution of school nurses unknown. Further, the competence of school nurses for this work also needs addressing in view of Brajkovich & Madison's (1986), Fahey & Cutting's (1988) and Goodeve's (1991) findings.

Consumer views

The limited empirical literature falls into three categories: children as consumers, parental expectations and teachers' perceptions of school nurses. McPherson & MacFarlane (1988) sought to gain an understanding of why teenagers ($n = 643$) make limited demands upon the health care system. Interestingly, only 1% considered themselves in poor health; however, this finding is confounded by a lack of definition as to what constituted good health.

Three-quarters of the sample suffered from headaches and had taken medicine in the previous 4 weeks, and a further third described having potentially important health problems. A surprising finding was the relatively small role that teachers and medical staff were viewed as having, with 86% of the sample claiming that they would first consult their parents over a health problem.

Fahey & Cutting (1992) also found some ambivalence about the school health service ($n = 90$) 'with the majority ... suggesting that medical inspections are best carried out by their GPs'. However, this survey, drawing upon a convenience sample of 16–19 years, identified a number of services which pupils viewed positively. For example, three-quarters of the sample supported the idea of health interviews. In contrast, weight and height measurement was considered unnecessary. Nash (1987) has claimed that there is little social distance between school nurses and children, although her empirical evidence is suspect and relies upon what she described as 'an informal sally among a group of school children' (sic) and even after a health care interview, Williamson (1992) found no significant increase ($n = 99$) in the likelihood of reference to a school nurse about a health problem. Indeed, there appears to be a significant image problem for health professionals working with children.

Parental views

The evidence of parental views is more substantial and draws upon several surveys. The desire for regular medical examination of primary school children is a consistent finding (Lucas 1980; Whitmore *et al.* 1982a,b; Cutting & Fahey 1987). This may require acknowledgement at a time when a selective approach is utilized. Such overwhelming desire for a system now replaced suggests either that parents have not been convinced of the merits of selectivity or that they had benefits which were not apparent in the cost-effectiveness analyses undertaken prior to the change of approach.

Parents also supported regular hygiene inspections of primary school children (Cutting & Fahey 1987). Fahey & Cutting (1988) also found that 89% of their non-randomized parental sample (*n* = 150) viewed regular medical examinations of secondary school children as necessary. Indeed, it is clear that what parents want is often very different from that which they receive from the health care services.

Finally, regarding health education, the parent survey suggested that 'the school nurse was not necessarily seen as the person who should teach'. Interestingly, a rather dated survey carried out by the HVA School Nurses' Group (1981) (*n* = 282) revealed a preference among school nurses for not having responsibility for medical examination and screening work (100%), as compared to a desire to undertake 'pre-school visits, home visits and health education' work (90.1%).

This apparent mismatch between consumers and providers needs to be addressed if the ideal of making services more responsive to consumers (DHSS 1986a) and client-centred, as advocated by the Cumberlege Report (DHSS 1986b), is to be realized. Perkins' (1989) study also highlighted the need to inform parents about every aspect of the school health service, together with their desire not only to be informed about screening events but also about the outcome of such examinations.

Teachers' perceptions

A lack of understanding of the current role of school nurses is also exemplified by the empirical evidence recording teachers' perceptions of the field of work. A very small survey of head teachers (*n* = 12) revealed that they held similar expectations to those of parents regarding the role of school nurses (Staunton 1983). They considered the main function of school nurses to be related to screening and the least important function included health education work.

These findings replicate the earlier work of O'Brien (1969). A general lack of understanding of what school nurses do was also highlighted by Hanson's (1987) survey of 46 teachers who perceived school nurses as both responsible for, and carrying out, screening and surveillance work (tasks enumerated on the questionnaire included vision testing, preparation for and assistance at school medicals, head inspections) in preference to teaching health education and advising teachers on health education.

Interestingly, there was a clear discrepancy between all the responses relating to the responsibilities of the school nurse and those relating to what 'the school nurse is seen to do'. The expectations of school nurses and the reality of their perceived performances varied from a discrepancy of 6%–37% on the itemized task list. A more recent study (Jones & Gordon 1992) has confirmed the low visibility of school nurses, with only a minority of the 78 teachers surveyed identifying the school nurse as the source of health information regarding pupils. Jones' (1992) survey similarly revealed a gap between head teachers' perceptions of the school nurse's role and observed school nurse activity, and there was clear evidence of poor communication between the head teachers and the school nurses.

While the school nurse is in an ideal position to act as a link between parents, teachers and other professionals (Hawes 1989), the degree to which nurses fulfil this potential is left to the individual practitioner. Indeed, the idiosyncratic performance of school nurses was revealed in part by the findings of Nash's (1985) survey of 25 school nurses in Hampshire, which found an enormous variation in the frequency of contact with other agencies:

'Those who made contacts, do so consistently. Those who did not relate, did not.

While practitioners perform their roles in such different ways, it is clear that outsiders or consumers will not be presented with a consistent image of the role of the school nurse, yielding the confusion recorded by Perkins (1989). Indeed, a major criticism levelled at the school health service in the UK is that it has failed to consult with parents, children, schools and local education authorities regarding its configuration of services (Audit Commission, 1994). If this is the case, it is not surprising that consumer views are generally negative.

School team

However, Holt's (1990b) appraisal pilot study in Southampton has suggested that both school nurses and teachers felt points of contact between them had been improved with the introduction of health care interviews in their area. Similar developments were reported to Wade *et al.* (1989) in their feedback session following 1 year of health care interviews for 13–14-year-olds in the Brighton Health District.

Nonetheless, evidence suggests that the full integration of nurses into the school team is not being realized but, as Carpenter (1985) has argued, such integration is essential if children are to benefit fully from the health services provided in our schools and this issue needs addressing urgently. Furthermore, the incorporation of children with special needs into mainstream schooling under the auspices of the 1993 Education Act makes the consideration of the issue of integration extremely critical.

Conclusion

In a climate of economic stringency, the school health service in the UK is under mounting pressure to demonstrate its usefulness and cost-effectiveness. It has long been recognized that the school health service has been dogged by a lack of understanding compounded by poor-quality information about what type of health service school children actually receive (National Children's Bureau 1987). Indeed, so scarce are data and evaluative research that Harrison & Gretton (1986) dubbed it 'the invisible service' and Roche & Stacey (1984, 1986, 1987, 1988) have consistently found school health service literature representing one of the smallest categories of entries in their overviews. In addition, the published papers included in their overviews are now overwhelmingly descriptive rather than analytical. This lack of empirical work may in part explain the absence of national policy guidelines, for it is clear that planners and managers have no data upon which to draw conclusions, a point which was acknowledged by Hughes (1988).

Project Health (HVA 1991) calls for major changes in the service with the accompanying survey of 381 school nurses claiming that their early intervention work made a major contribution to the health of school children in their care. However, while there is a lack of evidence demonstrating the cost-effectiveness of the service, health authorities may prefer to cut back upon the school health service rather than other services in an attempt to meet their financial targets (Jackson 1991).

The school health service is now almost 100 years old (Sadler 1991) but it is one of the most under-researched areas of health care provision. This review suggests that the service must be a priority area for research if practice and service delivery are to be cost-effective and benefit the health of school children, and the noble health targets of the British government's consultative document are to be realized (DoH 1991). Further, the Audit Commission (1994) has suggested that 'The school nurse is increasingly becoming the key professional involved', which re-emphasises the need for research to evaluate their effectiveness.

References

Audit Commission (1993) *Children First: a study of hospital services.* HMSO, London.

Audit Commission (1994) *Seen But Not Heard – coordinating community child health and social services for children in need.* HMSO, London.

Bailey, C. (1989) The developing role and training of the school nurse. *Health at School,* 5(3), 90–91.

Balding, J. (1992) *Young People in 1991.* Schools Health Education, University of Exeter, Exeter.

Baly, M.E. (1987) *A History of the Queen's Nursing Institute: 100 years, 1887–1987.* Croom Helm, Beckenham, Kent.

Bax, M. & Whitmore, K. (1989) Child health surveillance: a critique of Hall. *Health Visitor,* 62(7), 207–9.

Bone, M. & Meltzer, H. (1989) *The Prevalence of Disability Among Children: OPCS Surveys of Disability in Great Britain, Report 3.* HMSO, London.

Brajkovich, H.L. & Madison, R. (1986) A California school nurse credential survey. *Journal of School Health,* 56(10), 437–9.

Brand, C. (1980) Quite a challenge. *Nursing Times: Community Outlook,* December, 377–82.

Carpenter, M.J. (1985) Health care of the school child. *Nursing,* 2(39), 1167–70.

Challener, J. (1990) Health education in secondary schools – is it working? A study of 1418 Cambridgeshire pupils. *Public Health,* 104, 195–205.

Collis, J. (1985) Why educate school nurses? *Health Visitor,* 58(5), 123–4.

Cutting, E. & Fahey, W. (1987) What parents expect from primary school health services. *Health at School,* 2(9), 269–70.

Department of Health (1991) *The Health of the Nation* Cmnd 1523. HMSO, London.

Department of Health and Social Security (1976) *Fit for the Future: Report on the Committee on the Child Health Service* Cmnd 6684 (Chairman: Prof. S.D.M. Court). HMSO, London.

Department of Health and Social Security (1986a) *Primary Health Care: An Agenda for Discussion.* HMSO, London.

Department of Health and Social Security (1986b) *Neighbourhood Nursing – A focus for Care. Report of the Community Nursing Review* (Chairman: Mrs J. Cumberlege). HMSO, London.

Department of Trade and Industry (1989)*A Summary of Accidents in Education Institutions.* DTI, London.

Department of Transport (1990) *Road Accidents – Great Britain 1989.* HMSO, London.

Diamond, I.D., Pritchard, C., Choudry, N., Fielding, M., Cox, M. and Bushnell, D. (1988) The incidence of drug and solvent abuse among southern English normal comprehensive schoolchildren. *Public Health,* 102, 107–14.

Dickson, R.A. (1984) Screening for scoliosis. *British Medical Journal,* 289, 269–70.

Dobbs, J. & Marsh, A. (1985) *Smoking Among Secondary School Children in 1984.* HMSO, London.

Eckersall, S. (1985) The school nurse as educator. *Health Visitor,* 58, 289.

Education (Administrative Provisions) Act (1907). HMSO, London.

Education Act (1944). HMSO, London.

Education Act (1993). HMSO, London.

Essen, J. & Wedge, P. (1982) *Continuities in Childhood Disadvantage.* Heinemann Educational, London.

Fahey, W. & Cutting, E. (1988) What parents expect from secondary school health services. *Health at School,* 3(9), 272–4.

Fahey, W. & Cutting, E. (1992) Pupils' views of school nurses. *Community Outlook,* 2(3), 29–32.

Feuerstein, P. & Galli, N. (1983) Linking health screening to health education learning modules for elementary school students: a feasibility study. *Journal of School Health,* 53, 10–13.

Fixler, D.E. & Pennock, W. (1983) Validity of mass blood pressure screening in children. *Pediatrics,* 72, 459–63.

Fletcher, K. & Balding, J. (1992) *School Nurses do it in Schools!* Amalgamated School Nurses' Association, Huntingdon, Cambridgeshire.

Fothergill, N.J. & Hashemi, K. (1991) Two hundred school injuries presenting to an accident and emergency department. *Child: Care, Health and Development,* 17, 313–17.

Fyfe, J. & Ellerbroek, D. (1984) Colour vision defects and the school nurse. *Nursing Times*, 24 June, 48–9.

Goodeve, J. (1991) HIV/AIDS education: a study of school nurses; views of their role and an evaluation of two interventions in the school setting. Unpublished BSc dissertation, Department of Nursing Studies, King's College, University of London, London.

Graham, P.J. (1986) Behavioural and intellectual development. In Childhood Epidemiology (eds E.D. Alberman & C.A. Peckham). *British Medical Bulletin*, **42**(2), 155–62.

Gunatilleke, R. (1992). Outside the mainstream. *Primary Health Care*, **2**(10), 18–19.

Hall, D.M.B. (ed.) (1989a) *Health for All Children: A Programme for Child Health Surveillance*. Oxford University Press, Oxford.

Hall, D. (1989b) Ringing the changes in child-health. *Health Visitor*, **62**(8), 239–41.

Hall, D.M.B. (1989c) Health for all children and language testing. *Health Visitor*, **62**(12), 382–4.

Hall, D.M.B. (ed.) (1991) *Health for All Children*, 2nd edn. Oxford University Press, Oxford.

Hanson, L. (1987) No longer the nit lady. *Nursing Times*, **83**(22), 30–32.

Harrison, A. & Gretton, J. (eds) (1986) *Health Care UK: An Economic, Social and Policy Audit*. Policy Journals, Hermitage, Berkshire.

Hawes, N. (1989) School nursing in Norwich Health Authority. *Health Visitor*, **62**, 351–2.

Hawton, K. (1982) Attempted suicide in children and adolescents. *Journal of Child Psychology and Psychiatry*, **23**(4), 497–503.

Health Visitors' Association (1991) *Project Health*. HVA, London.

Health Visitors' Association School Nurses' Group (1981). What school nurses want: results of the school nurses' questionnaire. *Health Visitor*, **54**(4), 163.

Henderson, P. (1976) *The School Health Service*. HMSO, London.

Holliday, K., Carter, E. & Cardwell, E. (1984) The school nurse as a health educator. *Health Visitor*, **57**(6), 182–3.

Holt, H. (1990a) Southampton's health appraisal pilot study. *Nursing Standard*, **4**(15), 30–31.

Holt, H. (1990b) Health appraisal study. *Nursing Standard*, **4**(16), 26–7.

Huffod, B.A. & Lipnicky, S.C. (1987) Promoting self-responsibility: using the school nurse in a health awareness program for primary students. *Journal of School Health*, **57**(5), 195–7.

Hughes, J. (1988) *Changing School Health Services. 1. Current Debates*. King's Fund, London.

Hughes, J. & Gordon, P. (eds) (1988) *Changing School Health Services. 2. Two Case Studies*. King's Fund, London.

Interdepartmental Committee on Physical Deterioration (1904). *Report of the Interdepartmental Committee on Physical Deterioration* Cmnd 2175, vol. 1. HMSO, London.

Jackson, C. (1991) Turning back the clock. *Health Visitor*, **64**(5), 148–9.

Johnstone, J. (1986) What do school nurses do? *Health Visitor*, **59**, 363–6.

Jones, J. (1992). What teachers think. *Primary Health Care*, **2**(10), 12–14.

Jones, C. & Gordon, N. (1992) The school entry medical examination: what do teachers think of it? *Child: Care, Health and Development*, **18**, 173–85.

Jones, C., Batchelor, L., Gordon, N. & West, M. (1989) The preschool medical: an evaluation of this examination and its role in child health surveillance. *Child: Care, Health and Development*, **15**, 417–34.

Kelsall, J.E. & Watson, A.R. (1990) Should school nurses measure blood pressure? *Public Health*, **104**, 191–4.

Kennedy, F.D. (1988) Have school entry medicals had their day? *Archives of Disease in Childhood*, **63**, 1261–3.

Konje, J.C., Palmer, A., Watson, A., Hay, D. & Imrie, A. (1992) Early teenage pregnancies in Hull. *British Journal of Obstetrics and Gynaecology*, **99**, 969–73.

Larcombe, I. (1991) Back to normality. *Nursing Times*, 17 April, 68–9.

Latham, A. (1981) Health appraisal/surveillance by school nurses. *Health Visitor*, **54**, 25–7.

Law, J. (1989) Surveillance – shifting priorities. *Health Visitor*, **62**(5), 155

Lawson, A. & Rhode, D.L. (eds) (1993) *The Politics of Pregnancy: adolescent pregnancy and public policy*. Yale University Press, New York.

Leff, S. (1989) A comprehensive selective programme of health surveillance at school. *Public Health*, **103**, 425–84.

Lenderyou, G. (1993). A healthy alliance. *Primary Health Care*, **3**(3), 26–7.

Lucas, S. (1980) Some aspects of child health care: contacts between children, general practitioners and school doctors. *Community Medicine*, **2**, 209–18.

McMaster, R. (1984) Vision testing and the school nurse. *Health Visitor*, **57**(11), 331–3.

Macnab, I.F. (1987) Hypertension in schoolchildren: the case for screening. *Health Visitor*, **60**(11), 318–83.

McPherson, A. & MacFarlane, A. (1988) What teenagers think about their health. *Health Visitor*, **61**(6), 224–5.

Moon, A. (1987) Picture of health. *Nursing Times*, 7 January, 49–50.

Nash, W. (1985) The day they made contact. *Nursing Times: Community Outlook*, May, 14–16.

Nash, W.E. (1987) School-children as consumers – what are their health needs? *Health Visitor*, **60**(11), 387–8.

National Children's Bureau (1987) *Investing in the Future*. NCB, London.

National Health Service Act (1977). HMSO, London.

Nelson, M. (1989) The changing role of the school nurse within Worcester and District Health Authority. *Health Visitor*, **61**(11), 349–50.

Nietupska, O. & Harding, N. (1982) Auditory screening of school children: fact or fallacy? *British Medical Journal*, **284**, 717–20.

O'Brien, M.J. (1969) A nurse in school – why? *Nursing Clinics of North America*, **4**(2), 343–9.

O'Callaghan, E.M. & Colver, A.S. (1987) Selective medical examination on starting school. *Archives of Disease in Childhood*, **67**, 1041–43.

OPCS 1988) *General Household Survey*. DHSS, London.

OPCS (1993) *Population Trends 74*. HMSO, London.

OPCS Monitor (1989) *Death by Cause: 1988 Registration*. HMSO, London.

Perkins, E.R. (1989) The school health service through parents' eyes. *Archives of Disease in Childhood*, **64**(7), 1088–91.

Plamping, D., Thorne, S. & Gelbier, S. (1980) Children as dental health educators. *British Dental Journal*, **149**, 113–15.

Plant, M.A., Peck, D.F. & Samuel, E. (1985) *Alcohol, Drugs and School Leavers*. Tavistock, London.

Potrykus, C. (1990) The Hall Report: progress or a backward step? *Health Visitor*, **63**(1), 7–9.

Proctor, S.E. (1986) Evaluation of nursing practice in schools. *Journal of School Health*, **56**(7), 272–5.

Reid, D. & Massey, D.E. (1986) Can school health education be more effective? *Health Education Journal*, **45**(1), 7–13.

Riches, B. (1980) School nursing – a personal view. *Nursing Times: Community Outlook*, September, 250–55, 311.

Richman, S. & Miles, M. (1990) Selective medical examinations for school entrants: the way forward. *Archives of Disease in Childhood*, **65**, 1177–81.

Roche, S. & Stacey, M. (1984) *Overview of Research on the Provision and Utilisation of Child Health Services*. University of Warwick, Coventry.

Roche, S. & Stacey, M. (1986) *Overview of Research on the Provision and Utilisation of Child Health Services. Update I*. University of Warwick, Coventry.

Roche, S. & Stacey, M. (1987) *Overview of Research on the Provision and Utilisation of Child Health Services. Update II*. University of Warwick, Coventry.

Roche, S. & Stacey, M. (1988) *Overview of Research on the Provision and Utilisation of Child Health Services. Update III*. University of Warwick, Coventry.

Rona, R.J. & Chinn, S. (1984) The national study of health and growth: nutritional surveillance of primary school children from 1972–1981 with reference to unemployment and social class. *Annals of Human Biology*, **11**(1), 17–28.

Royal College of Obstetricians and Gynaecologists (1991) *Report of the Working Party on Unplanned Pregnancy*. RCOG, London.

Sadler, C. (1991) Schooled in health. *Nursing Times*, 5 June, 16–17.

Saffin, K. (1992) School nurses immunising without a doctor present. *Health Visitor*, **65**(11), 394–6.

Smith, G. & Fellner, I. (1985) Improving the uptake. *Nursing Times: Community Outlook*, June, 46, 48, 51.

Smith, G.C., Powell, A., Reynolds, K. & Campbell, C.A. (1989) The five year school medical – time for change. *Archives of Disease in Childhood*, **65**(2), 225–7.

Speight, A.N.P., Lee, D.A. & Hey, E.N. (1983) Underdiagnosis and undertreatment of asthma in childhood. *British Medical Journal*, **286**, 1253–6.

Squire, A. & Dowell, A.C. (1989) Paediatric surveillance –a calendar for change. *Health Visitor*, **62**(12), 382–4.

Stark, O., Peckham, C.S. & Ades, A. (1986) Weights of British and French children (Letter). *Lancet*, (8485), 856.

Staunton, P. (1983) Images of the primary school nurse. *Nursing Times*, 31 August, 49–52.

Staunton, P. (1985) In a class of their own. *Nursing Times: Community Outlook*, September, 6–8.

Stewart-Brown, S. & Haslam, M.N. (1987) Screening for hearing in childhood: a study of national practice. *British Medical Journal*, **294**, 1386–8.

Street, S. (1981) Supporting the school child with eczema. *Health Visitor*, **54**(9), 374–5.

Thurmott, P. (1976) *Health and the School*. Royal College of Nursing, London.

Tuke, J.W. (1990) Screening and surveillance of school aged children. *British Medical Journal*, **300**, 1180–82.

Turner, R. (1986) Healthcare goes back to school. *Health Service Journal*, 24 July, 992.

UKCC (1994) *The Future of Professional Practice – the Council's Standards for Education and Practice following Registration*. UKCC, London.

Vine, P. (1991) Ninety nine and counting. *Health Visitor*, **64**(5), 150–51.

Wade, J., Sudain, E. & Bennett, J. (1989) Health care interviews in secondary schools – a review of the first two years' experience in the Brighton Health District. *Public Health*, **103**, 467–74.

While, A.E. & Bamunoba, M. (1992) A study of children's contact with the school health service during the first six years of compulsory education. *Health Visitor*, **65**(2), 53–4.

White, D.G., Phillips, K.C., Pitts, M., Clifford, B.R., Elliott, J.R. & Davies, M.M. (1988) Adolescents' perceptions of aids. *Health Education Journal*, **47**(4), 117–19.

Whitmore, K. & Bax, M.C.O. (1990) Checking the health of school entrants. *Archives of Disease in Childhood*, **65**, 320–26.

Whitmore, K., Bax, M. & Jepson, A.M. (1982a) Health Services in primary schools: the nurse's role –1. *Nursing Times: Occasional papers*, **78**(25), 97–100.

Whitmore, K., Bax, M. & Jepson, A.M. (1982b) Health services in primary schools: the nurse's role – 2. *Nursing Times: Occasional Papers*, **78**(26), 103–4.

Whyte, E. (1984) Health begins at school. *Nursing Times*, 21 November, 40–41.

Williamson, T. (1992) Health care interviews by school nurses. *Health Visitor*, **65**(11), 402–4.

Chapter 5
An assessment of the value of health education in the prevention of childhood asthma

DOREEN M. DEAVES, *BA, MPhil, RGN, RHV*
Health Visitor, Gnosall Health Centre, Stafford, England

A research project, which looks at the value of health education in the prevention of childhood asthma, is described. The project was a controlled trial by a health visitor focused within the community. This exploratory research looked at three groups of children over a 2-year period, and compared the effect of: (1) individual health education, and (b) group health education. During the first year, two groups were active, one receiving individual health education, the other collecting data of the same type. During the second year, a third group was involved in health education sessions. The findings have been similar in both cases, in that both groups have demonstrated a good improvement in knowledge of asthma and its treatment. Through the active involvement of using a peakflow meter and diary records in the health education programme, both groups receiving health education have shown a significant improvement in the morbidity indicators related to night symptoms and restricted activities. The qualitative analysis of the research also highlighted the value parents of asthmatic children place on counselling. This research has provided the framework for the development of asthma care in a group practice.

Introduction

Asthma is one of the most common diseases of childhood (Anderson *et al.* 1983). An estimated 10% of children suffer from the condition. The introduction of new treatments does not appear to have made any impact on either the morbidity or mortality rates (Mellis & Phelan 1971; Burney 1987), and yet it is often said that asthma is preventable.

The extent to which specific health education programmes can help have been explored by a number of workers (Jones 1981; Clark *et al.* 1980, 1986; Littlewood 1984). The majority of evidence for the health education approach comes from the United States of America (USA) where controlled trials have produced evidence of decreases in morbidity and in the use of hospital services (Maiman *et al.* 1979; Fireman *et al.* 1981).

In the UK the research is more limited, and a study by Hilton *et al.* (1986) produced inconclusive evidence of a reduction in morbidity, but positive evidence for an increase in understanding of asthma and patient satisfaction.

Research motivation

The original motivation for this research came from a request to address the problem of prevention of asthma in children, by one of the doctors in the general practice to which I am attached as a health visitor. Health visitors are ideally placed to deal with this problem, using our expertise in health promotion, combined with the unique opportunity which the job offers for visiting children at home. The intention of this research was to look at the effectiveness and efficiency of the methods that could be employed in the prevention of childhood asthma.

Subjects

Two group general practices in Staffordshire agreed to take part in this research project, and identified the children in their practice who were diagnosed asthmatic and aged between 3–16 years of age. The practices were similar in population size, demographic and geographic structure. Sixty-four children were recruited to the study, 37 from each practice; they were assigned to group A or group B. One child was subsequently eliminated from group B because she suffered with cystic fibrosis. The children remained within their practice groups throughout the study, as it was not possible to randomize the groups because of anticipated difficulties with contamination of results.

Professional assessment

Professional assessment of the severity of each child's asthma was under-taken by one of the doctors in each group practice. This was done using defined criteria which were as follows:

(1) *Mild:* diagnosis made after consideration, child presents with a cough/ nocturnal cough or wheezy bronchitis which is managed with the use of occasional bronchodilators.
(2) *Moderate:* diagnosis well established, requires occasional admission to hospital/time off school. Treated with bronchodilators ± prophylactic treatments.

(3) *Severe:* requires frequent admission to hospital or out-patient follow up. Treated with bronchodilators plus prophylactic treatments plus systemic bronchodilators or cortisone. Included in this group are children with home nebulisers.

Method

Parents were sent letters of introduction, explaining the study, and inviting their participation. Those who agreed to participate were interviewed at home. The information recorded related to the child's present state of asthma, degree of morbidity, the duration of the condition, present treatment and the parents' knowledge of asthma and its treatment. The parents and children in group A were then introduced to the health programme.

The child's state of asthma was assessed and recorded; the children were taught to use a peakflow meter and keep diary records of asthma events. The parents were also given a short explanation of the mechanisms of asthma, and the action of the treatment which had been prescribed for their child. A package of written information was given to reinforce the explanation, and for reference. The parents of children in group B, following the interview, were asked if they would keep a record of asthma events for their children.

Both groups were involved in the research programme for 12 months. Since this is a long period of time, both groups were contacted at 3-month intervals in order to maintain motivation and answer any questions that might have arisen.

Further interviews

At the end of the first year, all participants were interviewed again. The information recorded included asthma morbidity, changes over the year, and the value of being part of a research programme. At this point all children in group B, who had suffered more than two attacks of asthma in the study year, were invited to continue with the research for a second year.

Ten parents accepted the invitation; their children then became members of study group C. These children were assessed and introduced to the peakflow meter and diary system of recording asthma events. This group was invited to attend group health education sessions, which were held in the evening at the local community hospital.

Analysis of results

The results of the interviews had been tested for significant differences using a *t*-test to compare groups A and B at the beginning and end of the study year. Groups B and C were compared at the start of the second year. Group C was tested at the beginning and end of the second year, to see if there were any differences as a result of health education. Qualitative analysis has been used, to look at the value of health education in those areas where statistical analysis is inappropriate.

Results

Groups A and B were similar at the beginning of the study; there were no significant differences between them with regard to age of diagnosis, present level of control or type of medication. There were no differences with regard to morbidity indicators, such as number of attacks, night symptoms, trigger factors, seasonal variations or interruptions to daily life (Table 5.1). The level of parental knowledge of asthma and its treatment was similar; so too was their opinion about health education received to date (Table 5.2).

The only significant difference between the groups at this stage was in the parents' assessment of the severity of their child's asthma ($P < 0.01$). Table 5.3 shows the numbers and categories associated with this result.

The doctor's assessment of severity shows no difference between the groups (Table 5.4).

Table 5.1 Comparison of morbidity in groups A and B at the beginning of the study (percentages in parenthesis).

Age of diagnosis	Group A ($n = 32$)	Group B ($n = 31$)
< 2 years	9 (29)	11 (35.4)
2–5 years	15 (46.8)	17 (54.8)
5–10 years	8 (25)	3 (9.6)
Good control	30 (93.75)	25 (86)
Type of treatment		
oral	10 (31.25)	10 (32.2)
inhaler	19 (59.3)	25 (86)
nebuliser	4 (12.5)	3 (9.6)
Number of attacks in previous year	97	134
Days lost from school	206	307
Night symptoms suffered	22 (68.75)	22 (70.9)
Trigger factors identified	14 (43.75)	15 (48.3)
Seasonal variations suffered	22 (68.75)	20 (64.5)
Interruptions to daily life regularly	5 (15.6)	4 (12.9)

Table 5.2 Parents' knowledge of asthma and health education at the beginning of the study (percentages in parenthesis).

	Group A	Group B
Good knowledge of asthma	18 (56)	14 (45)
Good knowledge of treatment	19 (59)	20 (64)
Action to prevent attacks	18 (56)	14 (45)
Parents said they had been given information		
verbally	25 (78)	20 (64.5)
written	7 (22)	12 (38.7)
other	1 (3)	3 (9.6)
Timing of information		
immediately	10 (31)	11 (35.4)
after a while	23 (72)	22 (71)

Table 5.3 Parents' assessment of severity.

	Mild	Moderate	Severe	Total
Group A	14	17	1	32
Group B	24	7	0	31
Total	38	24	1	63

$t = 3.57$, d.f. $= 61$, $P < 0.001$.

Table 5.4 Doctors' assessment of severity.

	Mild	Moderate	Severe	Total
Group A	10	16	6	32
Group B	9	17	5	31
Total	19	33	11	63

$t = 0.21$, d.f. $= 61$, NS.

Prevention

The first interview with groups A and B raised some interesting points, which are worth consideration in terms of prevention. Approximately 70% of parents were able to identify the factors that triggered an asthma attack in their child. When asked to name the trigger factors, animals, pollen, infection and exercise were identified frequently by both groups (Table 5.5).

Interestingly many more parents in group B identified emotion as a cause than in group A. Parents were asked if they did anything to prevent attacks of asthma; 18 (56.25%) parents in group A and 14 (45.16%) in group B said

Table 5.5 Trigger factors identified by parents.

	Group A	Group B
Animals	18	11
Pollen	17	10
Infection	13	16
Exercise	10	11
Emotion	2	14
House dust mite	9	10
Cigarettes	6	8
Smoke	4	6
Fog	5	6

they did. At the outset, parents who could describe asthma in terms of narrowing of the airways, with reference to inflammation and mucus production, were considered to have a good knowledge of asthma. The results show that 18 (56%) in group A and 15 (45%) in group B were considered to have a good working knowledge of asthma. With regard to treatment, the figures were slightly higher, with 19 (59%) in group A and 20 (64%) in group B demonstrating a good understanding of treatment, making the distinction between bronchodilator and prophylactic therapy.

Value of health education

The value of health education is the main feature of this research project, and parents were asked if they considered they had been given enough information about asthma, its prevention, treatment and care. Only 11 (34%) in Group A and 8 (25%) in group B felt they had been given enough information. The majority said the information they had been given was verbal, with seven parents in group A and 12 parents in group B saying they had received some written information. The most frequent information-givers were general practitioners.

Results at the end of the first year

There was no attrition of children from groups A or B during the first year of the study, but there were gaps in daily records, usually due to holidays or family crises. The results relate both to data collected, and the results of the final interview, which fall into one of three categories.

Morbidity indicators

The data collected by groups A and B related to: (a) number of attacks and days lost at school, and (b) night symptoms and restricted activities. There was no significant difference between the groups for number of attacks, or days lost at school (Figs. 5.1 and 5.2). The results related to night symptoms, and restricted activities, do show a significant difference between the two groups, at $P < 0.001$ (Table 5.6).

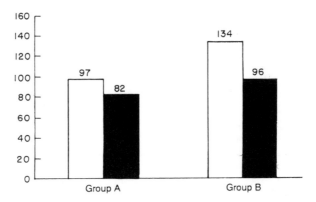

Fig. 5.1   Number of asthma attacks. ☐ = 1986–1987; ■ = 1987–1988.

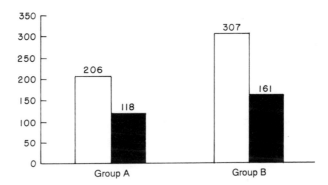

Fig. 5.2   Number of days lost at school or playgroup. ☐ = 1986–1987; ■ = 1987–1988.

Table 5.6   Morbidity in groups A and B at the end of the first year of the study.

	Group A (n = 32)	Group B (n = 31)
Number of attacks	82	96
Days lost at school	118	161
Night symptoms	69	121
Restricted activities	45	75

Knowledge of asthma and treatment

Parents in both groups were asked to describe asthma and its treatment; the results were assessed using the same criteria as in the initial interview. The two groups differed markedly, with the intervention group (group A) showing a high proportion of parents with good knowledge of asthma and treatment ($P < 0.001$) (Table 5.7).

Table 5.7   Parents' knowledge of asthma and treatment at the end of the study year (percentages in parenthesis).

	Group A ($n=32$)	Group B ($n=31$)
Good knowledge of asthma	31 (96.8)	16 (51.6)
Good knowledge of treatment	30 (93.75)	20 (64.5)

Parent satisfaction

Two-thirds of the parents said it was very valuable to use a peakflow meter and keep records (Fig. 5.3). Generally, the educational material was valued less by parents (Fig. 5.4). Although children in group B only kept records, they were asked whether this had been of any value. One-third said that it had been very valuable, and one-third said it had been no value at all (Fig. 5.5). Parents in group A said that using a peakflow meter and records were more helpful in prevention of attacks than written information (Figs 5.3 and 5.4).

Analysis of peakflow readings and diary records

The results of the peakflow readings and diary records of attacks were analysed in various terms which are: (a) related to the expected and observed

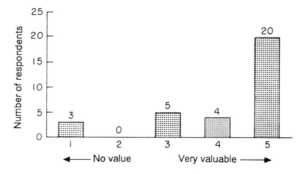

Fig. 5.3   Peakflow meter and diary records: group A.

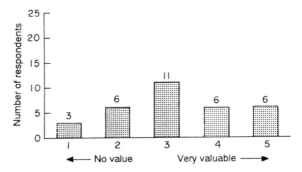

Fig. 5.4 Educational material: group A.

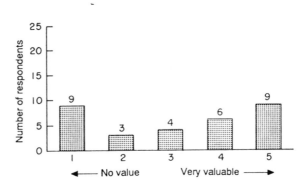

Fig. 5.5 Keeping diary records: group B.

values, and (b) variation related to the number and severity of attacks. Thirty of the 32 children in group A used a peakflow meter, and all kept diary records. The results are shown in Figs 5.6 and 5.7. The results show that some subjects wheeze with less than 20% variation in peakflow readings. The greatest variation of 50% or more occurred in those children described as moderate asthmatics.

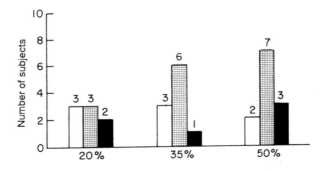

Fig. 5.6 Variation in peakflow readings. □ = mild; ▦ = moderate; ■ = severe.

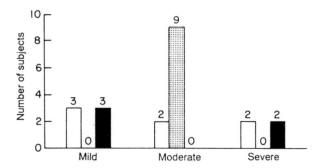

Fig. 5.7   Severity of asthma attacks. □ = mild; ▦ = moderate; ■ = severe.

Comparison between groups B and C

Ten parents accepted the invitation to continue with the study, although 23 children were eligible. Comparison at this stage revealed similarities and differences between the groups, which were:

(1) No differences between these groups in respect of any of the morbidity indicators, or parental knowledge of asthma and treatment (Table 5.8).
(2) Distinct differences in the areas that related to parents' perception of the situation (Table 5.9).
(3) Differences between the groups in the parents' assessment of severity of asthma ($P < 0.01$).
(4) Differences in parents' need for medical help, and parents' feelings about whether their child had got better or worse during the first year, and in the assessment of whether children had suffered more or less attacks than the previous year ($P < 0.01$) (Table 5.9).

From the results, it would appear that parents who volunteered to join group C had more to gain than those who did not volunteer.

Table 5.8   Difference between groups B and C at the beginning of the second year (percentages in parenthesis).

	Group B ($n = 21$)	Group C ($n = 10$)
Number of attacks	65	37
Days lost at school	108	53
Night symptoms	69	43
Restricted activities	44	31
Good knowledge of asthma	10 (47.6)	5 (50)
Good knowledge of treatment	12 (57)	9 (90)

Table 5.9 Parents' perception of asthma (percentages in parenthesis).

	Group B (n=21)	Group C (n=10)
Parents' assessment of severity		
mild	19 (90)	5 (50)
moderate	2 (9.5)	5 (50)
severe	0	0
Improvement in year		
much better	12 (57.1)	1 (10)
slightly better	8 (38.0)	4 (40)
remained the same	1 (4.7)	4 (40)
More or less attacks		
less attacks	11 (52.3)	1 (10)
same number	8 (38)	5 (50)
few more	2 (9.5)	2 (20)
many more	0	1 (10)
Parents' need for medical help		
needed less	13 (61.9)	0
needed more	8 (38)	10 (100)

Group C

All children in group C used a peakflow meter and kept diary records. One family dropped out of the study after 5 months. Results of the analysis at the end of the year showed:

Morbidity indicators

There were no significant differences between the groups in relation to number of attacks or days lost at school. But with respect to night symptoms and restricted activities there were significant differences ($P < 0.01$), which is similar to the first year (Table 5.10).

Knowledge of asthma and treatment

All parents at the end of the year were able to describe the mechanisms of asthma, and the mode of action of their child's treatment (Table 5.11).

Table 5.10 Group C at the end of the second year.

Morbidity	Year 1 (n=10)	Year 2 (n=9)
Number of attacks	27	23
Days lost at school	56	31
Night symptoms	43	20
Restricted activities	31	9

Table 5.11 Parents' knowledge of asthma and treatment (percentages in parenthesis).

	Year 1	Year 2
Good knowledge of asthma	5 (50)	9 (100)
Good knowledge of treatment	4 (40)	9 (100)

Analysis of peakflow readings and diary records

The results of peakflow readings in group C are similar to group A, with children described as moderate asthmatics, showing the greatest variation in peakflow readings and the highest number of moderate attacks.

Parent satisfaction

Again, all parents in group C felt that the use of a peakflow meter and records were more valuable than written information alone (Figs 5.8 and 5.9). Six parents found the group sessions extremely helpful; the other three

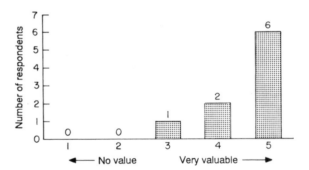

Fig. 5.8 Peakflow meter and diary records: group C.

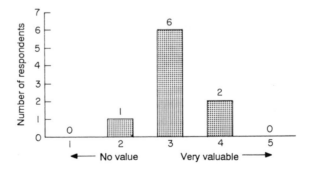

Fig. 5.9 Educational material: group C.

indicated that one would have been enough. Six of the parents said they felt more confident, and did not need to ask for medical help as frequently (Table 5.12). Seven parents appreciated the introduction of video information: they felt the inclusion of breathing and relaxation exercises particularly useful as this was an area often forgotten or undervalued by professionals.

Table 5.12 Parents' perception of asthma (percentages in parenthesis).

	Year 1 ($n=10$)	Year 2 ($n=9$)
More or less attacks		
less	1 (10)	6 (66.6)
same	5 (50)	3 (33.3)
few more	2 (20)	0
many more	2 (20)	0
Parents' need for medical help		
less help	0	5 (55)
as much help	10 (100)	4 (44.4)

The majority of parents (94%) had a great desire to be more involved with their child's care, and often expressed regret that they had not been given a diagnosis earlier, or been trusted with more information.

The discussion groups constantly highlighted the problem of receiving information from different people over time. Parents all felt they would value counselling a little while after the diagnosis had been made (i.e. 2–3 weeks), especially if that diagnosis had been given in hospital. Parents also expressed a need for continued education, in order to discuss issues as they arose.

Discussion

There are several significant findings from this research, which raise questions in relation to asthma education and the improvement in self-management.

The first relates to the parents' assessment of severity, which is both interesting and worrying. Looking comparatively at Tables 5.3 and 5.4, we see that there is a tendency for parents to assess their child's asthma less severely than do the doctors. Only one parent categorized her child as severe, and did so because she had been told that this was the case while the child was in hospital.

This finding supports some of the findings in studies related to deaths from asthma, which suggest that parents and sufferers have failed to appreciate the severity of the attack that has been fatal (Cushley & Tattersfield 1983).

Perhaps this failure to appreciate the severity of asthma is more generalizable among the lay populations than is realized by professionals. If that is so, then it is easier to see that parents and sufferers could fail to appreciate the severity of attacks. Acknowledgement of this factor may be important in the planning of future health education programmes.

Triggers

When parents were asked about prevention of attacks, approximately 70% were able to identify triggers for their child's attacks. The most commonly cited included pollen, animals and infection. More parents in group B thought emotion was a cause than in group A. When the doctors were asked what they thought were the most frequent causes of asthma, emotion was mentioned more often by doctors of group B children than group A children. Again, this response by parents may be influenced by information given to them, by people they respect.

One of the initial aims of this research was to improve knowledge of the mechanisms of asthma, and its treatment (Tables 5.2 and 5.7). At the outset, parents were a little more adept at describing treatment than understanding asthma. At the end of the study, groups A and C who had received health education differed significantly from group B in their knowledge of asthma and its treatment ($P < 0.001$).

Understanding the mechanisms of asthma, and the changes that occur as a result of bronchial reactivity, is an important prerequisite of understanding the effects of treatment (Rees & Price 1989; Gregg 1985). The two components cannot be separated, and the evidence tends to suggest that where people understand their medication, compliance with treatment will be higher than where they do not (Hay & Higenbottam 1987). This evidence would appear to be supported by the reactions of parents in this study, who said that, now that they understood the nature of preventive therapies, they would be more diligent and would encourage their children to use them.

Although there were no significant differences between the groups in the number of attacks suffered, or days lost at school, there was a reduction in numbers of both these findings for both groups (Figs 5.1 and 5.2). These findings may be a reflection of the increasing age of the children, since there do appear to be natural remissions with increasing age. They may also be a reflection of increasing interest in education; in reality, members of both groups may have become increasingly aware of self-management.

Night symptoms

The encouraging aspect of these results is that they do show differences in the morbidity indicators related to night symptoms and restricted activities.

Night symptoms are considered by most doctors to be a sign of poor control of asthma. To have shown a significant difference in night symptoms, and restricted activities, may indicate that health education can produce improvements in morbidity. To test this further, more intensive work would need to be done with larger numbers.

The findings of this study are similar to those of Hilton *et al.* (1986) in respect of knowledge and the main morbidity indicators, but suggest that there is some indication that education can influence morbidity.

Prevention of asthma is the fundamental aim of improving knowledge and treatment, and in this respect the approach to improving asthma is multifactorial. Although understanding what triggers an attack may form the basis of preventive action which could be undertaken by parents or children, in practice it is not always possible to use avoidance techniques.

This study programme introduced the use of a peakflow meter and records, in order to measure airway obstruction, and form a basis for prevention. Each child's peakflow was measured at the start of the study, and related to the expected value. The parents were given information about:

(1) The results of the reading.
(2) How to interpret the changes in peakflow readings.
(3) Assessing when to take action.
(4) What action to take in each circumstance.
(5) When to call a doctor.

From the analysis of the results (Figs 5.6 and 5.7), it can be seen that the number of attacks in relation to variation in peakflow readings is greatest in those children described as moderate asthmatics. This could suggest that they are the ones who need more attention, and have the most to gain. The results in general reflect the clinical picture accepted by most practitioners in that asthma is depicted as a very variable condition and needs individual attention in relation to each sufferer; and cannot be standardized into groups beyond the simplest levels. This also reinforces the suggestion that self-management requires a great deal of understanding by the sufferer and supportive information from the professional.

Peakflow

Analysis of the records revealed that in four instances actions taken by parents as a result of reduced peakflow readings may have prevented the onset of an attack. Two of these instances were related to children in the severe category and therefore the most vulnerable to severe, and possibly fatal, attacks. This finding, although small, may be crucial. It suggests that parents have gained confidence in their own abilities to take action, and this has proved successful.

For the children in groups A and C, the effectiveness of treatment, or the lack of it, may well have been highlighted by the regular use of a peakflow meter. This type of monitoring may well lead to changes in treatment, or the mode of delivery of treatment. The regular use of peakflow meters and records had been of greater value to parents than educational material alone. If this is the case, it may also lead to a more active involvement in the management of the condition by parents and children.

Analysis of the findings in relation to this study has not been confined to statistical analysis alone. There are more complex issues involved, which demonstrate the confidence and coping skills of the parents and children, or the limitation placed upon those coping skills. The limitations on individual coping skills may arise from lack of information. The enabling powers of the health professionals may also be at fault. Parents said they felt that they were not trusted with information. Other factors may be within the parents, families or children themselves.

Health education attempts to provide information in order to enhance these coping skills. The manner in which the information is offered, and the status of the health professional involved, may improve trust and enable parents to cope better with their child's asthma.

Parents said, at the beginning of the study, that the majority of health education information given to them had been in relation to causes, prevention and treatment, and was given verbally. Parents considered infection, pollen and animals to be the most frequent triggers for attacks in their children. The doctors identified atopy as the major factor, but thought infection played a significant part in children's asthma, and 50% said they were liberal users of antibiotics.

Parents' questions

The questions uppermost in parents' minds seemed to be:

(1) Why had they not been told sooner that their child had asthma?
(2) When do children 'grow out of it'?
(3) What needs to be done in severe attacks?

In this study, all the doctors said they would consider more than one episode of wheezing as potential asthma. Eight out of 10 said they would tell the parents as soon as possible, which tended to be after the second or third episode of wheezing.

Some children will 'grow out of asthma': the evidence seems to suggest that approximately 70% will be free of wheeze at 21 years old (Price 1984; Rees & Price 1989). The difficulty tends to be in relaying this to the parents who may perceive a general statement as a promise that this will definitely happen to *their* child. This makes professionals cautious, but can create uncertainty in parents.

One of the barriers to the improvement of confidence in the management of asthma seemed to be the extent to which parents were confused about the information they had received. Mainly, they were not always sure that the information was complete. Some parents felt there was a fear on the part of the medical services to trust them with information and treatment. They said this affected the trust they had in the doctors.

Over-anxious parents did not seem to be very evident to the researcher, but the basic lack of understanding seemed to add to the anxieties of parents. Parents felt very strongly about the need to clarify information, and needed someone with whom to explore their feelings. This led to the suggestion that counselling after the diagnosis is made, especially when that diagnosis is made in hospital, would help to resolve some of these problems.

Parents felt strongly that this counselling should ideally take place at home, at best 2–3 weeks after diagnosis. This time interval, they felt, would give them time to come to terms with the diagnosis. Timing was considered to be most important because educational information given too soon could be lost by the emotional state of the parents. As time passed, parents then felt they needed to be able to ask questions, and that there was someone available from whom to seek information, without feeling they were consuming doctors' valuable time. The ideal person to provide this information seems to be a member of the nursing profession.

Research outcomes

This research has looked at the value of health education in the management of childhood asthma. The health education programmes have been based on the active involvement of parents and children in the process. It has been successful in improving parental knowledge and satisfaction, and has shown significant improvements in some of the morbidity indicators. The benefits of the programme to parents has been an improvement in confidence in the management of their child's asthma. This is very important considering the variability of asthma and the fact that it can be a life-threatening condition.

The empirical findings of this study suggest that:

(1) The regular use of a peakflow meter and diary records, along with explanations of the results and actions to be taken, are an important part of improving parents' confidence.
(2) Parents should be offered the opportunity of counselling at home, within a few weeks of diagnosis, and this approach should be incorporated into the management of childhood asthma.

(3) Health education programmes incorporate information related to the severity of asthma suffered by the individual child.

Health education

The findings of this study have shown that health education can make improvements in some morbidity indicators, namely those of night symptoms and restricted activities. This may be where the 'tip of the iceberg' begins to melt. Further studies, incorporating larger numbers, are needed in order to demonstrate whether these findings can be applied to larger populations.

Research based development of nursing practice

This is an example of a situation in which the original motivation for research into the prevention of childhood asthma has led directly to the development of asthma care for children in Gnosall. The research findings have provided a model of prevention and health education with maximum nurse involvement, and have helped develop a protocol of holistic care in which medical and nursing care are complementary to each other. The medical model of care is no longer the dominant feature.

In practice, the asthma clinic, run by a health visitor, is a regular weekly feature. All clinic attenders have a full assessment of their asthma, which is recorded on an information card. Treatment and inhaler techniques are reviewed and a self-management programme is planned. Self-management programmes use peakflow measurements and diary records to monitor the percentage change in peakflow readings and the recurrence of symptoms.

Fig. 5.6 shows that there is no consistent percentage change for all sufferers, at which symptoms recur. This means that management can only be planned on an individual basis. The usual advice given is to reverse the fall in peakflow using bronchodilators, with a subsequent increase in prophylaxis for a few days, resuming the maintenance programme when the peakflow measurement returns to normal. The parents and/or children are given specific advice to deal with attacks and deteriorating symptoms.

Regular review of the self-management programmes allows for development and the changing pattern of their condition, as a considerable number of children do 'grow out of asthma'.

All newly diagnosed children are offered the opportunity for a home visit, to provide the counselling that is felt to be missing by parents. Asthma is often considered to be an environmental disease (Burney 1988), so this provides the opportunity to look at the primary preventive aspects and to give information on control or prevention of allergens in the home.

Asthma care in Gnosall includes group meetings, which create an opportunity for parents to discuss their concerns and reinforce the education of their children, in an informal way, with professional help available if needed.

Conclusion

Practical research experience is a valuable tool in the evaluation of practice, because it teaches us to be analytical. Asthma lends itself to quantitative audit, based on the improvement in peakflow measurements and morbidity symptoms, but we must not forget that quality of life is a prime concern.

Often with asthma patients, being symptom free equates to improved quality of life, but so does better understanding of the condition and the feeling of being in control. Nurses must take every opportunity to help asthmatic children and parents take proper control of a condition which is potentially life long and life threatening.

Acknowledgements

This study was undertaken for a Master of Philosophy degree. I would like to say thank you to my director of studies, Professor Jane Robinson at Nottingham University, and my supervisors of various stages, Ms Cynthia Clamp and De Chris Brannagan at Birmingham Polytechnic, and also to Dr Patty Mazelan for the statistical advice; to Sean Hilton for his advice, and to the general practitioners in both participating practices, and to all families; to Mid-Staffordshire Health Authority to whom I am grateful for being allowed to conduct the research, and for the research scholarships. I would also like to thank Maws Ltd and the Health Visitors Association for their Community Project award.

References

Anderson, H.R., Bailey, P.A., Cooper, J.S., Palmer, J.S. & West, S. (1983) Morbidity and school absence caused by asthma and wheezing illness. *Archives of Disease in Childhood*, **58**, 777–84.

Burney, P.G. (1987) Asthma mortality: England and Wales. Evidence for a further increase in 1974–84. *Lancet*, **ii**, 323–6.

Burney, P. (1988 Why study the epidemiology of asthma? *Thorax*, **43**, 425–8.

Clark, N.M., Feldman, C. & Freudenberg, N. (1980) Developing education for children with asthma through self management behaviour. *Health Education Quarterly*, **7**(4), 278–97.

Clark, N.M., Feldman, C.H., Evans, D., Duzey, O., Levinson, M.J., Wasilewski, Y. *et al.* (1986) Managing better: children, parents and asthma. *Patient Education and Counselling*, **8**, 27–38.

Cushley, M.J. & Tattersfield, A.E. (1983) Sudden death in asthma: discussion paper. *Journal of the Royal Society of Medicine*, **76**, 662–6.

Fireman, P., Friday, G.A., Gira, C., Vierthaler, W.A. & Michaels, L. (1981) Teaching self-management skills to asthmatic children and their parents in an ambulatory care setting. *Paediatrics*, **68**(3), 341–8.

Gregg, I. (1985) Quality of care in General Practice: a challenge for the future. *Family Practitioner*, **2**, 94–100.

Hay, I.F.C. & Higenbottam, T.W. (1987) Has the management of asthma improved? *Lancet*, **ii**, 609–11.

Hilton, S., Sibbald, B., Anderson, H.R. & Freeling, F. (1986) Controlled evaluation of the effects of patient education on asthma morbidity in general practice. *Lancet*, **i**, 26–9.

Jones, R.T.S. (1981) Management of asthma in the child aged under 6 years. *British Medical Journal*, **282**, 1914–16.

Littlewood, M. (1984) Asthma – a support group. *Nursing Times*, **80**, 40–42.

Maiman, L., Green, L.W., Gibson, C. & McKenzie, E.J. (1979) Education and self treatment by adult asthmatics. *JAMA*, **241**, 1919–22.

Mellis, C.M. & Phelan, P.D. (1971) Asthma deaths in children: a continuing problem. *Thorax*, **32**, 29–34.

Price, J. (1984) Asthma in children: diagnosis. *British Medical Journal*, **288**, 1666–8.

Rees, J. & Price, J. (1989) *ABC of Asthma*, 2nd edn. *British Medical Journal*. Cambridge University Press, Cambridge.

Chapter 6
Familial inflammatory bowel disease in a paediatric population

GLORIA JOACHIM, *RN, MSN*

Assistant Professor, School of Nursing, University of British Columbia, Vancouver, British Columbia, Canada

and ERIC HASSALL, *MBC, FRCP(C)*

Associate Professor, Paediatrics, and Head, Division of Paediatric Gastroenterology, British Columbia Children's Hospital, Vancouver, British Columbia, Canada

Familial aspects of inflammatory bowel disease (IBD) were assessed as part of an age and sex matched case control study of 91 children with IBD and 131 controls. The prevalence of IBD in family members of the children was studied, the affected side (mother's side or father's side) of the family was documented and the type of inflammatory bowel disease was traced among relatives. Data were collected from children in out-patient clinics at a large urban tertiary-care facility. All family data were verified with the affected relatives and/or their physicians. The children with IBD (the cases) had significantly ($P = 0.0000385$) more IBD in their families than the controls. Among all children with IBD in their family, IBD was found significantly ($P = 0.0073$) more often on the mother's side of the family than on the father's side. Patterns of disease varied within families. A mixture of ulcerative colitis and Crohn's disease was found within families. The implications of the findings are discussed. Directions for prevention, screening, early intervention and further study are given.

Introduction

Inflammatory bowel disease (IBD) is a chronic ideopathic long-term disorder. IBD includes Crohn's disease and ulcerative colitis. Despite a lack of knowledge about causation, it has been accepted that there is an increased prevalence of IBD among the relatives of IBD patients. A variety of studies have surveyed patients regarding the presence of disease in their families. Most studies to date have concentrated on adult IBD patients. Ascertaining the diagnoses of parents or grandparents of adult children is a difficult task. The question of accuracy of the data arises.

More information about familial IBD would help to clarify risk factors, assist with prevention and screening and might shed light on the mode of transmission of this disease. As part of a case control study of children with IBD, familial patterns of IBD were studied. All family diagnoses were verified. This chapter describes the prevalence of IBD in family members of children enrolled in the study, documents the affected side of the family, and traces the diseases that appear among the relatives.

Background

Calkins & Mendeloff (1986) state, 'The greatest risk for IBD seems to occur in those who share the most genes with the propositus'. A high family prevalence of IBD was first noted in the 1970s (Singer *et al.* 1971; Lewkonia & McConnell 1976). A rate of familial IBD between 5% and 40% has continued to be documented (Mayberry *et al.* 1980; Weterman & Peña 1984; Calkins & Mendeloff 1986; Lashner *et al.* 1986; Gilat *et al.* 1987; Monsen *et al.* 1987; Haug *et al.* 1988; Farmer 1989; Küster *et al.* 1989; Roth *et al.* 1989; Orholm *et al.* 1991). The only studies that reported a low familial occurrence were one conducted in Japan (Yoshida & Murata 1990), where the appearance of IBD is recent, and one site (Mediterranean area) of a multi-site paediatric study (Gilat *et al.* 1987).

Data sources

Data for the above studies were collected in a variety of ways. Sources included written questionnaires independently filled out by the probands, personal interviews with probands and record reviews. Of the cited works, only a few stated that the data regarding family members with IBD were verified with the family member, medical records or the physician caring for the identified family member (Lashner *et al.* 1986; Küster *et al.* 1989; Roth *et al.* 1989; Orholm *et al.* 1991). If data were not verified, the potential for inaccuracy resulted.

Patterns of familial IBD varied. Gilat *et al.* (1987), in an international paediatric study, found no predominant parent–child relationship. Farmer (1989) concluded that the most frequent familial pattern association is sibling/sibling followed by first cousins – a horizontal rather than vertical relationship.

Other studies have reported that siblings have the highest incidence of IBD among first-degree relatives (Lewkonia & McConnell 1976; Mayberry *et al.* 1980; Weterman & Peña 1984; Monsen *et al.* 1987; Roth *et al.* 1989), although Orholm *et al.* (1991) found no difference in the relative risk among parents, children and siblings.

In two studies a trend was found for relatives to have the same disease as the patient when Crohn's disease was the diagnosis. However, this trend was absent when the diagnosis was ulcerative colitis (Hammer *et al.* 1968; Roth *et al.* 1989). Others (McConnell 1980; Calkins & Mendeloff 1986) found the diseases mixed in families.

Unfortunately, the literature that documented the lineage of the family where IBD occurred was not found. While family groupings were described, they were always referred to as relatives rather than specifically stating whether on the mother's or father's side. Then the data are mixed, and gaps exist in our knowledge of familial patterns.

Methods

Objectives

Based on the literature and results of an earlier pilot study (Joachim 1991), a large study was designed to gather information about genetic aspects of IBD. A paediatric population was selected because of the short disease history, relative ease of accessibility of relatives (grandparents, aunts and uncles) compared to an adult population, presence of a parent to help with accurate recall and the assumption that families of newly diagnosed children (within 2 years of diagnosis) might have acquired great awareness of IBD among family members as they searched for information about the problem.

It was deemed important to test not only the prevalence of IBD among family members, but to trace the presence of IBD according to the side of the family. Moreover, the authors were able to examine whether only one type of IBD exists within a family or if the two types occur simultaneously within families.

Study population

A study of 91 children with IBD (the cases), 80 otherwise healthy children with acute orthopaedic injuries (control group A) and 51 children with another chronic disease – cancer – (control group B) was conducted.

Data collection

All children were recruited through out-patient clinics in a large tertiary-care facility. The children lived in Vancouver and throughout the province of British Columbia. All were from roughly the same catchment area. All children were between 6 and 17 years old, and were diagnosed as having their respective conditions within the previous 2 years. The IBD cases were diagnosed by standard endoscopic and radiologic tests. The control children with orthopaedic injuries and cancer were officially diagnosed in their respective clinics.

All IBD children and a parent who visited the gastroenterology clinic between January 1989 and April 1991 were approached and asked to participate. Informed consent was obtained and a personal interview conducted. Controls were age (within 2 years) and sex matched to the cases. Children and a parent were approached and asked to participate during a clinic appointment.

Standardized data were collected from each patient and parent pair by a nurse research assistant. A family pedigree was taken according to side of the family. Fig. 6.1 shows the data requested.

Number of siblings with Crohn's disease (CD)   ☐ (enter actual number 0–9)

Number of siblings with ulcerative colitis (UC)   ☐ (enter number 0–9)

Does your father or anyone on his side of the family have inflammatory bowel disease?

Father		Aunt		Uncle		Cousin		Grandma		Grandpa	
☐	☐	☐	☐	☐	☐	☐	☐	☐	☐	☐	☐
CD	UC	CD	UC	CD	UC	CD	UC	CD	UC	CD	UC

(Enter the actual number of each: for example, if two aunts have CD and one has UC, enter   ☐   ☐)

Does your mother or anyone on her side of the family have inflammatory bowel disease?

Mother		Aunt		Uncle		Cousin		Grandma		Grandpa	
☐	☐	☐	☐	☐	☐	☐	☐	☐	☐	☐	☐
CD	UC	CD	UC	CD	UC	CD	UC	CD	UC	CD	UC

(Enter the actual number of each)

Fig. 6.1 Familial data collected from the cases and control.

Database creation

After the data were collected, those records positive for familial IBD were copied into a new database, named Study Gen. In addition to housing records, the Study Gen database also sorted familial data according to the mother's side and father's side of the family. Table 6.1 shows a part of the Study Gen database.

The parent of each patient with a positive family history was contacted to obtain the name, address and telephone number of the ill family member.

Table 6.1   Part of the Study Gen database.

	CD	UC	CD	UC
Rec Num 107		Group Code 100		Diagnosis 1
Sex: F	Father		Mother	
Parent	0	0	0	0
Aunt	0	0	0	0
Uncle	0	0	0	0
Cousin	0	0	0	1
Grandma	0	0	0	0
Grandpa	0	0	0	0
Rec Num 111		Group Code 100		Diagnosis 1
Sex: F	Father		Mother	
Parent	0	0	0	1
Aunt	0	0	0	1
Uncle	0	0	0	0
Cousin	0	0	0	0
Grandma	0	0	0	1
Grandpa	0	0	0	0

The named family member was then contacted by G.J. (principal investigator) to confirm the diagnosis. In some instances the family member confirmed the diagnosis through a detailed report of symptoms and naming either Crohn's disease or ulcerative colitis as well as naming a gastroenterologist who diagnosed the illness. In other cases, permission was obtained to contact the gastroenterologist or family physician, who then confirmed or disclaimed the diagnosis of IBD. A new database – Study Gen Verif – was created. The new database contained only confirmed familial IBD.

The new database was examined to determine whether or not IBD appeared more frequently on one side of the family than the other, and to track the type of IBD found in the case, control and their relatives.

Results

Prevalence of inflammatory bowel disease among relatives

Data were obtained from 222 children each with a parent present. There were 91 cases and 131 controls. In the Study Gen database, 48 subjects reported a positive family IBD history. Of these subjects, 32 had Crohn 's disease, three ulcerative colitis, seven had an orthopaedic injury and six had cancer.

Upon validating the data with the named relative and his/her physician, numerous errors were detected. Among the cases with Crohn's disease there were nine errors, that is, nine relatives could not be confirmed as having IBD. Reasons for not confirming the diagnoses included recall errors: relatives remembered to have IBD actually had diverticulitis, Yersinian enterocolitis, parasites, irritable bowel syndrome, or had not officially been diagnosed with IBD. Among the three cases with ulcerative colitis, one relative had not been officially diagnosed. Among the seven orthopaedic patients (control group A), who named a relative with IBD, three families could not be located, and one recall error exists: the named relative did not have IBD. All others were confirmed. Of the cancer children (control group B), all six reports of IBD were confirmed.

Twenty-five IBD cases – 23 with Crohn's disease and two with ulcerative colitis – had confirmed relatives with IBD. Three orthopaedic controls and six cancer controls also had confirmed relatives with IBD. A chi-square calculation was done with the verified data (Table 6.2).

Table 6.2   Prevalence of familial inflammatory bowel disease among the cases and controls.

	IBD	Controls
Positive family history	25	9
Negative family history	66	119
Totals	91	128

Odds ratio = 5.01
95% CI (2.09–12.85)

	χ^2	*P*-value
Uncorrected	16.95	0.0000385
Yates corrected	15.42	0.0000859

The records of the three orthopaedic patients who could not be located were deleted, leaving 128 controls. There were significantly ($P = 0.0000385$) more family members with IBD among the IBD cases than among the controls. The odds ratio (OR) = 5.01 with 95% confidence limits = 2.09, 12.85.

Side of family of affected relatives

The cases and controls were pooled to determine if a difference existed in terms of side of the family of the affected relatives. Two cases and one control subject had IBD on both sides of the family. These three subjects were excluded from the side of family portion of the analysis. Of the remaining 31 subjects with IBD verified in the family, 21 (62%) had IBD on the mother's side and 10 (29%) on the father's side. There were no instances of affected siblings. A test of proportion shows the difference to be significant ($P = 0.00732$).

When testing the side of the family of the relatives and comparing them with the children who had no IBD in their families, the results remained significant ($P = 0.042$).

Disease of family members

Some children had more than one family member with IBD. Of the 23 children with Crohn's disease, there were 13 relatives with ulcerative colitis and 12 relatives with Crohn's disease. The two children with ulcerative colitis had two relatives with Crohn's disease. The three children with orthopaedic injuries had one relative with ulcerative colitis and two with Crohn's disease. The six children with cancer had six relatives with ulcerative colitis and one with Crohn's disease. Table 6.3 shows characteristics of the 34 children with IBD confirmed in the family.

Table 6.3 Characteristics of the 34 children with inflammatory bowel disease (IBD) confirmed in the family (all children are between the ages of 6 and 17).

	Sex of child		IBD on mother's side	IBD on father's side	IBD on mother's and father's side
Diagnosis	M	F			
Crohn's disease	12	11	18	7	2
Ulcerative colitis	2	0	1	1	
Orthopaedic injury	2	1	1	2	
Cancer	3	3	4	3	1

Discussion

Findings of this study show that 25 (28%) of the cases had relatives who also had IBD. This finding was significantly different from that of the controls. IBD among both the cases and controls was found significantly more frequently on the mother's side of the family than on the father's side. There was an absence of IBD among siblings. There seems to be no clear relationship between the diagnosis of the case and his/her relative(s). A mixture of Crohn's disease and ulcerative colitis exists among family members. This supports the findings of Calkins & Mendeloff (1986).

Limitations

Some limitations exist that may have an influence on the results. Although data were collected from a large tertiary-care facility, where the majority of children with IBD are seen, and children come from all over the province of British Columbia, there are children with IBD who are seen in their own doctor's offices. While this study certainly includes the majority of children with IBD in the catchment area, it does not include all of them. However, there is no reason to believe that the missed cases were specifically either family history or side of family affected to measure the exact number of children seen for IBD because out-patient visits were not counted and coded in the province.

There may be a lack of awareness about IBD among relatives, particularly when families are dispersed. Hence, the number of relatives with IBD may be under-reported. Finally, since the highest incidence of IBD occurs in the 15–25 year age group (Whelan 1990), the decision to conduct a paediatric study of children between 6 and 17 years of age limits the number of cases in the study. Expanding the study to include an adolescent and young adult population would certainly increase the numbers of cases.

Recall bias was clearly demonstrated when 10 IBD cases and a parent incorrectly identified a relative as having IBD. Only one recall error existed among the controls, but unfortunately three control families could not be located to confirm or disprove the identification of IBD in their families. Recall bias was addressed by contacting relatives and their physicians.

When considering the preponderance of IBD on the mother's side versus the father's side of the family, the possibility of familial awareness again occurs. Since most of the patients were interviewed with a mother only present, it is possible that the mother was more aware of her own history than the father's and, therefore, could have under-reported the father's background.

Strengths

Strengths of the study include the single interview which minimized the potential for losing cases and controls over time when follow-up is required. Uniform diagnostic criteria were used since all IBD patients were recruited from a single clinic when the same diagnostic procedures are followed. The data collected were standardized and all data were collected by two interviewers trained by G.J. (principal investigator).

Selection bias was considered when out-patient clinics were chosen as the vehicle for recruitment. In-patient hospital studies miss those patients seen only in clinics, but during the course of the 15 months of data collection, all in-patients eventually became out-patients thereby maximizing the sample size.

Conclusions

As was expected, 28% of the cases had IBD in the family and the cases had significantly more IBD than the controls. This rate did not differ from the literature. The verification process ensured as much accuracy as possible. The absence of siblings with IBD is conspicuous and may be due to the young age of the patients. It would be interesting to follow these cases in the future to see how many siblings develop IBD. It would also be of interest to follow the controls with a positive family history to see if they or their sibling develop IBD.

Of the controls, more from control group B (cancer) reported IBD in the family (7.5%) than control group A (orthopaedic) (5.5%). Could it be that there are some similarities between the two chronic disease groups?

Most of the recall error among the cases was due to inaccurate recall about the relative's diagnosis. Most of those relatives were found to have other inflammatory type conditions of the gastrointestinal tract, such as diverticulitis, Yesinia enterocolitis and irritable bowel syndrome. If all of the inflammatory conditions were grouped together instead of limiting the criteria for IBD to Crohn's disease and ulcerative colitis, the rate of bowel disease among the cases would be much greater. Perhaps there is a common element, and some families are at risk for all kinds of bowel disease. The presence of several different gastrointestinal disorders in a family would support this idea.

Mother's side of the family

There were significantly more instances of IBD on the mother's side of the family. Could IBD be genetically linked to the mother's side, or was the father's side underreported? Repeating this study, but interviewing the cases and controls with their fathers instead of mothers, might yield interesting results.

The question remains: is the presence of IBD due to heredity or environment? There have been only a few studies reporting IBD that developed among non-blood relatives in the same house (Whorwell *et al.* 1978; Farmer *et al.* 1980; McConnell 1980). A study of family members who were separated at birth would help to generate hypotheses.

Is it possible that there are two types of IBD: one caused by genetic factors and the other by environmental factors? Further studies of family pedigree and environmental factors would confirm or disprove this thought.

Implications

The implications of obtaining more knowledge about familial IBD are clear. Prevention and family planning could be undertaken appropriately.

Screening for high-risk individuals or families could be available. Early intervention might prevent some of the costly long-range complications for the affected individuals, their families and society.

Acknowledgements

This study was funded by the British Columbia Health Research Foundation. The authors thank Drs Sam Sheps and Martin Schechter, Department of Health Care and Epidemiology, University of British Columbia, for their ongoing help and guidance with this project.

References

Calkins, B.M. & Mendeloff, A.I. (1986) Epidemiology of inflammatory bowel disease. *Epidemiologic Reviews*, **8**, 60–91.

Farmer, R.G. (1989) Study of familial history among patients with inflammatory bowel disease. *Scandinavian Journal of Gastroenterology*, **170** (Suppl.), 64–5.

Farmer, R.G., Michever, W.M. & Mortimer, E.A. (1980) Studies of family history among patients with inflammatory bowel disease. *Clinics in Gastroenterology*, **9**, 271–8.

Gilat, T., Hacohen, D., Lilos, P. & Langman, M.J.S. (1987) Childhood factors in ulcerative colitis and Crohn's disease: an international cooperative study. *Scandinavian Journal of Gastroenterology*, **22**, 1009–24.

Gilat, T. & Rozen, P. (1979) Epidemiology of Crohn's disease and ulcerative colitis: etiologic implications. *Israel Journal of Medical Science*, **15**, 305–8.

Hammer, B., Ashurst, P. & Naish, J. (1968) Diseases associated with ulcerative colitis and Crohn's disease. *Gut*, **9**, 17–22.

Haug, K., Schrumpf, E., Barstad, S., Fluge, G. & Halvorsen, J.F. (1988) The study group of inflammatory bowel disease in Western Norway. *Scandinavian Journal of Gastroenterology*, **23**, 517–22.

Joachim, G. (1991) The epidemiology of inflammatory bowel disease in children: a pilot project. *Journal of Advanced Nursing*, **16**(7), 794–9.

Küster, W., Pascoe, L., Purrmann, J., Funk, S.S. & Majewski, F. (1989) The genetics of Crohn's disease: complex segregation analysis of a family study with 265 patients with Crohn's disease and 5,387 relatives. *American Journal of Medical Genetics*, **32**, 105–8.

Lashner, B.A., Evans, A.A., Kirsner, J.B. & Hanauer, S.B. (1986) Prevalence and incidence of inflammatory bowel disease in family members. *Gastroenterology*, **91**, 1396–1400.

Lewkonia, R.M. & McConnell, R.B. (1976) Familial IBD – heredity or environment? *Gut*, **17**, 235–43.

McConnell, R.B. (1980) Inflammatory bowel disease: newer views of genetic influences. In *Developments in Digestive Disease* 3 (ed. J.E. Berk), pp. 129–37. Lea & Febiger, Philadelphia.

Mayberry, J.F., Rhodes, J. & Newcombe, R.G. (1980) Familial prevalence of inflammatory bowel disease in relatives of patients with Crohn's disease. *British Medical Journal*, **1**, 84.

Monsen, U., Brostrom, O., Nordenvall, B., Sorstad, J. & Hellers, G. (1987) Prevalence of inflammatory bowel disease among relatives of patients with ulcerative colitis. *Scandinavian Journal of Gastroenterology*, **22**, 214–18.

Orholm, M., Munkholm, P., Langholz, E., Nielsen, O.H., Sorensen, T.I. & Binder, V. (1991) Familial occurrence of inflammatory bowel disease. *The New England Journal of Medicine*, **324**, 84–8.

Roth, M.P., Petersen, G.M., McElree, C., Vadheim, C.M., Panish, J.F. & Rotter, J.K. (1989) Familial empiric risk estimates of inflammatory bowel disease in Ashkenazi Jews. *Gastroenterology*, **96**, 1016–20.

Singer, H.C., Anderson, J., Fisher, H. & Kirsner, J.B. (1971) Familial aspects of inflammatory bowel disease. *Gastroenterology*, **61**, 423–30.

Weterman, I.T. & Peña, A.S. (1984) Familial incidence of Crohn's disease in the Netherlands and a review of the literature. *Gastroenterology*, **86**, 449–52.

Whelan, G. (1990) Epidemiology of inflammatory bowel disease. *Medical Clinics of North America*, **74**, 1–11.

Whorwell, P.H., Eade, O.E. & Hassenbocus, A. (1978) Crohn's disease in a husband and wife. *Lancet*, **ii**, 186–7.

Yoshida, Y. &.Murata, Y. (1990) Inflammatory bowel disease in Japan: studies of epidemiology and etiopathogenesis. *Medical Clinics of North America*, **74**, 67–90.

Chapter 7
Parents' experience of coming to know the care of a chronically ill child

MARY D. JERRETT, *RN, MSc, EdD*

Associate Professor, School of Nursing, Queen's University, Kingston, Ontario, Canada

The family is the primary source of care for a chronically ill child, and it is the parents who must manage the child's illness on a daily basis. This qualitative study was undertaken to investigate the ways in which 10 two-parent families of children with juvenile arthritis experience their child's illness. In this chapter the theme of coming to terms with the management of the illness and what it entails for the parents is examined. The data provide evidence of how the parents learn, and their efforts and experience of learning to care for the child on a daily basis. This is a complex process and includes the different phases the parents experience as they move through the learning process. The findings suggest that the parents learn the child's care and make adjustments to the demands of managing the child's illness in a way that works best for them.

Purpose of the research

The purpose of this research was to investigate the ways in which parents of children with the chronic illness juvenile arthritis experience their child's illness. More particularly, it focused on the parents' perspective of how they manage the experience. The family is the primary source of care for a chronically ill child, and parents must manage the illness on a daily basis. For parents this invariably increases the amount of physical care, and heightens the emotional and mental effort that must be devoted to child care. The significance of the problems associated with the care of the chronically ill child is underscored by the demands made on the family (Patterson 1988).

The importance of a broader understanding of parents' perceptions of the child's illness management, and adjustments that must be made in order to accommodate the demands of the experience, has been emphasized in the literature (Anderson 1981; McCubbin 1984; Knalf & Deatrick 1986; Anderson & Elfert 1989; Deatrick & Knalf 1990; Kodadek & Haylor 1990; Whyte 1992). Chronic childhood illness, however, remains a major challenge for nurses as they conceptualize family caregiving and involve families in their child's care.

Source of learning for parents

In this chapter, the process the parents go through as they come to terms with managing the child's illness is interpreted as a source of learning. A learning metaphor is used to examine their perceptions of the experience and guide the interpretive process. A fundamental assumption underlying this study is that the care of an ill child is a challenge for parents, and to live such an experience is to learn. From this premise follows yet another assumption, which is that for parents the child's illness management is best learned through active involvement, personal discovery, and that parents are motivated towards this end. Thus, it follows that the parents' experience of caring for their chronically ill child offers a view of the processes by which they learn to manage their child's illness, and affirms the experience and efforts of the parents to learn.

Conceptual perspective

The experience of illness needs to be considered within the context of its meaning for the individual and for the family. 'Illness as a human experience of loss or dysfunction has a reality all its own' (Benner & Wrubel 1989). Thus, to understand the meaning of illness for the person afflicted, and in this study the parents, it is necessary to hear the parents' account, their perceptions of the situation, their day-to-day life, including the physical work involved, and the stress and emotional responses. In addition to fulfilling the usual duties and obligations of being parents, they are now expected to meet the new needs arising from the illness. This constitutes a severe disruption to the ordinary continuity of family life as previously understood.

Typically, when a child gets sick the parents contact someone in the health care system, and frequently seek out a physician for help. The doctor will assess the symptoms and prescribe a treatment. The focus of the treatment is on the symptoms that are indicators of the disease and on the specific therapeutic interventions required. Further, it is assumed that most children will get well or at least improve if the parents do what is expected of them – in other words, if they follow 'the orders'. Yet, the experience for the parents cannot be reduced merely to a scientific account of the disease, to a prescribed treatment; it needs to be considered within the context of their actual lives. That is, their subjective experience is fundamentally important not just because it involves a personal reassessment of objective reality, but because lived experience is reality (Kestenbaum 1982). Thus, there are two ways to think of the child's illness, that is, two ways of knowing about the particular experience. First, there is the actual disease of pathology to reckon with, and second, there is the perspective of how the disease and treatment affect the parents' role and family life.

These two different views of the illness experience can be conceptualized as two kinds of awareness (Polanyi 1962). He describes 'focal' awareness and 'subsidiary' awareness as being two types of knowing that are mutually exclusive. Focal awareness involves knowing about the object or technical aspects of the experience, while subsidiary awareness contributes to the quality of the focal event. Subsidiary awareness occurs at all levels of consciousness, while focal awareness is always at the conscious level only.

Phenomenological perspective

The phenomenological perspective was used in this study. Deeply rooted in this approach is the assumption that the researcher must understand the meaning of the experience from the frame of reference of the study participants. The aim of the researcher is to consider the experience as it is lived, 'to capture the relational quality of the person in the situation' and to be attentive of the particular situation (Benner 1985). This approach involves obtaining a description of the experience as it is lived from the perspective of the participants in order to provide a deeper understanding of the experience (Omery 1983).The aim is to study 'persons, events and practices in their own terms'; to articulate meanings and an understanding of the lived world of the participants (Benner 1994). Thus, the phenomenological approach, as used in this study, is concerned with the description of the experience of the parents involved, in order to understand more deeply and to make explicit their experience through interpretation. Understanding refers to the establishment of meaning and the term interpretation denotes 'the process of bringing to understanding' (Palmer 1969).

Experience is viewed as a source of human significance, and this involves others accepting it as it is perceived by the individuals concerned (Colaizzi 1973). Furthermore, experience is not static, formed once and for all; it is interactive and changes over time. That is to say, our understanding of experience is shaped by our being in a certain context that has meaning for us, and by our ability to consider the situation in terms of its meaning for the particular individual (Benner 1985). Therefore to reveal the experience of the participants in this study, the focus is on the accounts they gave of themselves and of their situation. The care of a chronically ill child is a particular experience and each parent is an individual with a unique perspective; yet there are patterns that can be determined from each person's account and meanings that are common to all.

Study participants

The participants in this study were parents, in two-parent families, of children with juvenile arthritis, an illness that is non-life threatening. It is also an illness in which a parent is likely to be involved with the child's care. In many studies involving parents, only the mothers participate because they are assumed to be responsible for the child's day-to-day care. However, both parents in two-parent families share a common world with the child. To understand the reality of that world requires hearing from both. Therefore, fathers' perceptions are included in this study. Nineteen parents from 10 families participated. Of these, both parents in nine of the families were interviewed separately in their homes. One father was not willing to be interviewed.

There are advantages to be gained from interviewing both the mother and the father. The first is that two accounts are obtained rather than just one. Hence, it seems plausible that a more reliable picture of the experience may emerge as issues in one interview are confirmed or acknowledged by the other. Further, with two accounts, one version may supplement information not given in the other. Most of the interviews lasted approximately 2 hours. The mothers, as primary care-givers, were interviewed two or three times, while the fathers were interviewed once, with the exception of one who was interviewed twice.

Data collection and analysis

The interview was the method of data collection; the initial interview was deliberately exploratory and wide-ranging, a method frequently adopted in qualitative studies. The intention was to discover the parents' experience through listening to their stories by allowing them to speak for themselves. As the study progressed, and areas of special concern surfaced, the interviews became more focused. All the interviews were tape recorded and later transcribed.

Interpretive analysis is an ongoing process and is carried out concurrently with the interviews. This approach provides an understanding of subjective meaning, and entails calling upon information uncovered through the descriptive process. The parents' description of their experience is turned into a text through transcription, and the focus of the interpreter is to discover common meaning and to achieve understanding. It is necessary, then, to read and reflect upon the transcription of the interviews in order to gain insight and understanding of the parents' experience. This means returning to the tapes and transcripts again and again and exploring them from different angles.

This is a process that involves going from understanding parts to understanding the whole; going from words to larger units of thought in order to discover the themes of meaning embedded in the parents' accounts. With thematic analysis the themes, or patterns, are considered the commonalities of experience around which interpretation occurs (Polkinghorne 1983). Furthermore, 'common themes, common meanings and even common personal concerns are expected in a study of human beings who have common cultural backgrounds and are in common situations' (Benner & Wrubel 1989).

It is necessary to ensure that the themes or patterns identified by the researcher capture what is expressed by the parents; this entails discussing the interpretations with each participant, and constructing meaning with them (Anderson & Elfert 1989). As Benner (1985) points out, themes can be systematically and vigorously validated by experts as well as those who are living out the meanings presented in the interpretation. However, the conceptual formulations from the data are determined by the researcher (Anderson & Elfert 1989).

Results

The successful management of a child's chronic illness hinges on the parents being able to provide the prescribed care once the child is discharged from hospital. It is often taken for granted by health care professionals that the parents will do what is expected of them, that they will carry out the prescribed treatment regime. The parents in this study regarded their situation with subsidiary awareness; the illness experience and their interpretation of the situation were based on the conviction that the family held responsibility for the child's care. Hence, while the parents tended to focus on the subsidiary factors related to their focal problems, they learned to manage the care of their child with juvenile arthritis.

The interpretation presented here deals only with the theme of coming to know the illness management, and what it entails for the parents. There were other themes or commonalities of experience such as the experience of uncertainty and the parents' images about the siblings that will not be discussed. Coming to terms with their new reality and coming to know what is involved in caring for their chronically ill child extended for the parents over a period of several stressful years. Interpretation of the patterns of learning embedded in their experience is presented as a learning process in this study. Specific meanings are considered in each phase of the experience, as they moved from being merely reactive to becoming proactive learners.

Initial response – turmoil and confusion

There were important differences between the care parents were required to give a healthy child, as opposed to one with juvenile arthritis. In addition to the normal parental tasks, there was now the child's therapy to contend with. To fit into the day were exercises that involved painful stretches of the joints, usually distasteful medications to be given several times, splints to be applied to arms, legs and neck at night, trips to the physiotherapist, as well as the frequent appointments with health professionals. The child's therapy became an indelible and inescapable part of the parents' reality.

From the parents' accounts, it was evident that central to their initial reaction was confusion and emotional turmoil. They all at first felt unable to cope with what was happening to their child. Feelings of anger and devastation were universal responses to the anguish they experienced. The anger could be directed at almost anyone – the doctor, God, each other. The parents expressed their feelings in familiar terms that they found frustratingly insufficient to describe the extent of their emotions. As one said: there were 'no words'; their experience was outside the bounds of normal language and their idea of child rearing. She summed up her response in this way:

> 'I have the typical reaction ... it's too bad you have to use normal words like shock, devastation, anger; but those are the words you have to use.'

The parent's anger, sadness and feelings of helplessness were lived meanings, as were the conflict, tension and confusion they felt surrounding this new reality. As one mother explained:

> 'You go through feelings of anger or sometimes sadness; you go through the whole thing. The first year was just dreadful, it was a tempest. Nothing seemed to fit, everything was in a turmoil; you are so emotional.'

During this period of confusion and turmoil, the parents' emotional responses were viewed as markers, part of the shift in perspective which helped to open up possibilities as they began to make links between feelings and experience. Attending to feelings offered the parents an opportunity to develop new options for coping and new understanding. Hence, emotions were an essential part of coming to terms with the changes in their parenting role as they submitted to managing the new caregiving activities. Such feelings were considered to be the meanings, lived out by the parents, as they learned to manage the child's illness.

Struggling to know

The parents' descriptions of the child before the onset of the illness were viewed within the frame of old ways of knowing. Each parent saw their 'past' child from an individual unique perspective that, in turn, informed their coming to a different, new view of the child. The parents were now expected to take on an unfamiliar role, to carry out the distinctive activities involved in caring for a chronically ill child. Most did not feel prepared to do this. This reaction was often accompanied by feelings of being overwhelmed, complicated by a lack of information about the illness. As one mother pointed out:

> 'I have never heard of children having arthritis, and this is what really frightened me very much. I just didn't know anything and I assumed many things that really scared me, like she will be in a wheelchair, things like that. It's not like that, but that's how little we knew... It wasn't until after a lot of perseverance that we got information...'

The parents' subjective interpretation of the situation and their ability to manage the illness were often at odds with what the health care professionals expected of them. And this, in turn, increased conflict and confusion for them, and served to highlight their sense of isolation. Coming to terms with the prescribed therapy in particular, often proved to be a considerable struggle. To cause their children pain was opposed to the parents' natural instincts. For example, one mother described her anxiety about the therapy as a 'nightmare'; she despaired of doing it every day, and did not want to do what was expected of her.

For the parents, the need to manage the child's illness often placed them in a context in which their past understanding seemed no longer relevant; familiar features of their situations were no longer meaningful. However, their reactions filtered through their values, beliefs and expectations associated with child care. Little by little, as their bewilderment was redefined, more order emerged. As the parents became more confident, they moved away from simply reacting. They began to accept that managing their child's illness on a daily basis involved doing things differently from the past.

A different way of knowing

Once the parents' efforts were directed toward managing the child's prescribed therapy, it shaped how they experienced their situation. There were demands on their time, different demands from those they used to have. Thus, a schedule or routine provided the context in which the experience could be understood – it framed the experience and opened the door to new possibilities.

All the parents acknowledged the need to control time and the value of becoming organized. There was only a finite amount of time, and the work of caregiving was normally time-bound. Therefore, to control time itself became part of controlling the caregiving activities. They developed schedules and worked diligently at being organized. According to one mother whose child's illness management required more and more time:

> 'What I've tried to do is keep it really scheduled. In a sense that really

helped me. And I would say that I am really not an organized person and I like to be spontaneous; I think that's really my nature, but I found it really helped me to be organized.'

Through re-organization and working out a schedule, the parents were able to carry out their family responsibilities. The re-allocation of tasks was often stressful, but eventually the parents felt more capable. They found that their energies and attention were refocused once they had worked out a routine. In general, they were more responsive to doing the therapy once they had a schedule and had modified their past ways of knowing. Having a schedule gave them greater control of time. This resulted in positive feelings which, in turn, became part of their approach to the caregiving. This different way of knowing their circumstances was a more competent and certain knowing. They tried to maximize their potential and make sense of their situation, including the time-consuming and painful therapy. According to one mother:

'I think it's pretty good right now ... our days are full from morning till night, we do the therapy twice a day. It took me a long time to realize that unless she had her therapy she wasn't going to get any better, and even though she hurts at the time, after she felt a hundred percent better. You see, we have moved a long way...'

All of the parents admitted to life being more structured, and with this change, they seemed to discover new meanings in the understanding of their situation. The caregiving – or what they often referred to as 'the routine' – became part of their every day reality. Thus, the caregiving not only involved the activities with the child, but also the re-organization of self.

Taking charge

The parents eventually had a perspective that transcended the day-to-day distress of the child's illness management. Their world was reshaped as the care-giving activities became integrated into family life. Included also was the valuing of the complexities as they came to realize that the caregiving was not a straight forward process. The amount of control exerted by individual parents varied. With regard to the child's care, there were those things that were within the parents' control and some that were not. For example, to have the final word about the child's medication was often perceived as being within their control. There were times when the parents refused suggested changes in medication or took considerable time before they agreed. As one parent pointed out:

'When it comes to trying new drugs, we take our time and find out everything we can. As parents, I think that is what we have to do ... we have to make the final decision ... and if they [the doctors] don't agree with it, well you know, that's up to them, but she is our child.'

Other parents' accounts of how they behaved with health professionals had a great deal to do with their taking charge. As one parent noted:

'We don't necessarily accept what the doctor says as being God-given law ... we'll challenge it if there is a basis for challenge.'

Being able to challenge medical authority was thus instrumental in helping the parents acknowledge their ability to control or have input into decisions affecting their child. It was re-assuring to be part of the decision-making process; being involved facilitated better information exchange. As a father noted: 'Parents bring something special to the decision – the personal element, versus the scientific part.' The parents listened to and valued the expertise of the professionals, but also felt that they themselves had their own expertise based on what they had lived through.

With the growth of self-confidence they became more involved and, in turn, felt able to impose some meaning on their ability to affect change. They acknowledged their understanding of the child's best interests. Among parents there was a movement towards self-direction which included a sense of being able to take charge and manage the child's illness on a day-to-day basis. Acquiring this perspective took time, but was clearly present with six of the families.

Discussion

The findings highlight the patterns of learning embedded in the parents' experience as they lived through the events and activities surrounding the care of their chronically ill child. The illness altered the perception of their role and all went through considerable difficulty in grasping the meaning of their new reality. The parents all suffered varying degrees of tension, emotional turmoil, and contradictions around the lack of fit between past ways of knowing and the present circumstances. Benner & Wruble (1989) suggest that 'emotions allow the person to be engaged or involved in the situation', to be linked with the lived situation – which, in this study, were the meanings lived out by the parents.

An integral part of the meaning of the experience for the parents was judged to be an understanding of its nature, as they came to know what was expected of them. This was the phenomenon that the parents were involved in shaping as they learned to manage the child's illness, saw the possibilities inherent in the situation, gained some expertise and came to an understanding of what was required. Personal meaning arose from experience which individual parents interpreted within their own frame of reference.

For the parents, engagement and involvement in the child's care enabled them to draw on resources that eventually helped them to handle many demanding situations. They learned first hand about the possibilities inherent in their own particular circumstances and they developed an understanding of the experience that was rooted in their own frame of reference. This became their new reality which evolved from living with the child and managing the illness on a daily basis. Learning from experience was fundamental to understanding the care-giving for the parents; it was a form of practical knowledge or experience knowing (Schön 1983; Benner 1984; Benner & Wruble 1989).

The learning that occurred from their experiencing the caregiving moved from an early struggle to know, to a more competent, if at times uncertain, knowing. Hence, through experience, the parents learned to manage their particular situation, became familiar with the care their child required, and acquired new skills and strategies. Their inner struggle and the experiences they moved through as they came to understand how to care for their child were crucial to the learning process. Thus, the learning process became one that acknowledged and valued what the parents lived through, with its attendant joy and suffering.

Complexity

The complexity of the parents' experience was evident in their responses. There were times when the caregiving was truly distressing, yet there were times when it accorded them a certain satisfaction. Certainly, the restraints, regret and anguish they felt should surprise no one. This was particularly so for the mothers because they bore the brunt of the work; their own needs often became ancillary. However, like the parents in the study by Kodadek & Haylor (1990), it was clear that over time the parents learned to provide care in ways that seemed to work for them, and they were continually involved in shaping their particular experience. Although there were individual differences, there were also similarities, with some parents doing better than others in meeting the caregiving challenge and coping with the child's illness.

Conclusion

In conclusion, this study employed the concept of experiential learning to guide the interpretive process. It followed the phenomenological tradition that stresses the importance of understanding caregiving from parents' perspectives, and was concerned with the development of an interpretation of their way of being in the world.

The caregiving experience opened parents of children with juvenile arthritis to learning on many levels, as they struggled to make sense of their circumstance. As this study found, the child's chronic illness altered the parents' world. With their previously healthy child the parents knew their role and were accustomed to a particular child. With their ill child the situation was altered, they experienced considerable difficulty in grasping the meaning of their new reality, the meaning of providing care for their child. Yet, as the primary caregivers they were expected to implement complex treatment plans.

A noteworthy finding in this study was the ability of the parents to eventually develop expertise in their child's illness management. To assume responsibility for the caring work helped them to be more in control, and affirm their own way of knowing. For the parents the process of coming to know the child's illness was based on the practical knowledge that came from the experience of actually caring for the child. These parents challenged the widely held assumption that the family is a passive recipient of 'expert' advice.

Although parents' contribution to the health care system is considerable, this study suggested that their relationship with health professionals was far from ideal. Similar to parents in another study, they viewed the health care system as both a resource and a constraint (Ray & Ritchie 1993).

The findings from this study underscore the need for nurses to examine their practice as it relates to family behaviour patterns and responses, and to develop skills to negotiate conflict situations. Nurses must demonstrate an awareness of the experience the parents are living as they struggle to know the child's illness management. We need to ask questions which will illuminate this process.

Nurses need to further develop their assessment skills and direct attention at strategies for supporting the family with its unique caregiving needs (Wright & Leahey 1990). This includes helping families to find ways to use the health care system to their greatest advantage. Nurses must open the way to improved relationships between the family and the nurse; a model that means shared understanding and views the parents as partners involved in shaping their own role as caregivers. Further study is needed in order to examine more specifically how nurses function with families as they confront the arduous experience of managing their child's chronic illness.

References

Anderson, J.M. (1981) The social construction of the illness experience: families with a chronically ill child. *Journal of Advanced Nursing*, **6**, 427–34.

Anderson, J.M. & Elfert, H. (1989) Managing chronic illness in the family: women as caretakers. *Journal of Advanced Nursing*, **14**, 735–43.

Benner, P. (1984) *From Novice to Expert*. Addison-Wesley, Menlo Park, California.

Benner, P. (1985) Quality of life: a phenomenological perspective on explanation, prediction, and understanding in nursing science. *Advances in Nursing Science*, **8**(11), 1–14.

Benner, P. (1994). The traditional skill of interpretive phenomenology in studying health, illness and caring practices. In *Interpretive Phenomenology* (ed. P. Benner). Sage, London.

Benner, P. & Wrubel, J. (1989) *The Primacy of Caring*. Addison-Wesley, Menlo Park, California.

Colaizzi, P.F. (1973) *Reflection and Research in Psychology*. Kendall Hunt, Dubuque.

Deatrick, J.A. & Knafl, K. (1990) Management behaviors: day-to-day adjustments to childhood chronic illness. *Journal of Pediatric Nursing*, **5**(1), 15–22.

Kestenbaum, V. (1982) The experience of illness. In *The Humanity of the Ill: A Phenomenological Perspective* (ed. V. Kestenbaum), pp. 3–38. University of Tennessee Press, Knoxville.

Knalf, K. & Deatrick, J. (1986) How families manage chronic conditions: an analysis of the concept of normalization. *Research in Nursing and Health*, **9**, 215–22.

Kodadek, S. & Haylor, M. (1990) Using interpretative methods to understand family caregiving when a child is blind. *Journal of Pediatric Nursing*, **5**(1), 42–9.

McCubbin, M. (1984) Nursing assessment of parental coping with cystic fibrosis. *Western Journal of Nursing Research*, **6**(4), 407–10.

Omery, A. (1983) Phenomenology: a method of nursing. *Advances in Nursing Science*, **5**(2), 49–63.

Palmer, R.E. (1969) *Hermeneutics*. Northwestern University Press, Evanston, Illinois.

Patterson, J. (1988) Chronic illness in children and the impact on families. In *Families in Trouble Series: volume 2, Chronic Illness and Disability* (eds C.S. Chilman, E. Nunnally & F. Cox). Sage, Newbury Park, California.

Polanyi, M. (1962) *Personal Knowledge*. University of Chicago Press, Chicago.

Polkinghorne, D.E. (1983) *Methodology for the Human Science*. State University Press, Albany, New York.

Ray, L.D. & Ritchie, J.A. (1993). Caring for chronically ill children at home: factors that influence parents' coping. *Journal of Pediatric Nursing*, **8**(4), 217–26.

Schön, D.A. (1983) *The Reflective Practitioner*. Jossey-Bass, San Francisco.

Whyte, D.A. (1992) A family nursing approach to the care of a child with a chronic illness. *Journal of Advance Nursing*, **17**, 317–27.

Wright, L.M. & Leahey, M. (1990) Trends in nursing of families. *Journal of Advanced Nursing*, **15**, 148–54.

Chapter 8
Preparing children and families for day surgery

MARY-LOU ELLERTON, *RN, MN*
Associate Professor, School of Nursing, Dalhousie University, Nova Scotia, Canada

and CRAIG MERRIAM, *BA, MPA*
Director of Distance Education Programming at Henson College, Dalhousie
University, Halifax, Nova Scotia, Canada

The increasing use of ambulatory care settings for children's surgery
places more responsibility on parents for psychological preparation
of children for surgery and for their post-operative care. This
chapter describes the evaluation of a pre-admission programme to
prepare children between the ages of 3 and 15 years, and their
families, psychologically for day surgery. Seventy-five families
comprised the study sample, 23 in the programme group and 52 in
the non-intervention group. The programme focused on familiarizing families with the physical and procedural components of day
surgery through a videotape of a family in a naturally occurring day
surgery situation, a tour, and a hospital play session. Fewer children
and parents in the programme group reported high anxiety levels
while awaiting surgery. Children and parents with previous surgical
experience reported higher levels of pre-surgical anxiety than inexperienced families. Families identified physicians and day surgery
nurses as primary sources of information and rated the nurses
highest in their satisfaction with information received. Implications
for practice, particularly for meeting the needs of young children
and out-of-town families, are discussed.

Introduction

The use of ambulatory health care services continues to rise consistent with
federal and provincial restraint in health care funding. Same-day surgical
admissions have, in many instances, reduced hospital admission time from a
few days to just a few hours. However, the responsibility for preparing
children for same-day hospital stays rests largely on parents, many of whom
are anxious themselves and have uncertain expectations about the hospitalization and their role in helping their child manage the experience. Nurses in

ambulatory care settings describe many difficulties in providing sufficient information and psychological support to families admitted for same-day surgery.

The adverse effects of hospitalization on young children are well known to health care providers. Studies of hospitalized children have revealed more symptoms of psychological upset than in well children, as well as more fears and lower levels of self-esteem (Sides 1977; Ahmadi 1985; Abbott 1990). Post-hospitalization upset, including anxiety and aggression, sleep anxiety, fear of separation from parents, and apathy, have all been reported in children in response to a hospital experience (Vernon *et al.* 1966; Thompson 1985). The results of intervention studies which utilize preparation strategies suggest that psychological strategies can be effective in reducing children's pain and anxiety (Melamed & Siegel 1975; Men & Zastowny 1982; Lunch 1994).

Stressful factors eliminated

The introduction of day surgery for minor surgical procedures has eliminated many of the stressful factors associated with a conventional hospital experience. Day-surgery patients remain in close proximity to their parents for almost the entire duration of their hospitalization and have to manage fewer new experiences and encounters with strangers. Nevertheless, unfamiliar experiences associated with a hospital encounter of any sort can be distressing, especially to very young children. Discharge of the child from hospital within hours of surgery is also associated with increased parental responsibility for early post-operative care.

Much of the research in children's health care over the last decade has focused on methods of preparing children and families for hospital experiences and medical procedures. Preparation programmes which use procedural and sensory information, coping models, and play with hospital equipment have been associated with increased knowledge and less anxiety in children undergoing surgical procedures (Johnson *et al.* 1975; Meng 1980; Roberts *et al.* 1981; Patterson & Ware 1988; Stewart *et al.* 1994). The day-surgery programme at the Izaak Walton Killam Hospital for Children (IWK) was developed for its consistency with the philosophy of family-centred care adopted by the hospital and for its response to the needs for families in day surgery for information and support.

The study

The purpose of this study was to evaluate a pre-admission programme to prepare children and families psychologically for day surgery.

Method

The following research questions were investigated.

(1) What are the effects of the pre-admission programme on children and parents' anxiety before and after surgery?
(2) Does the programme have an effect on parents' satisfaction with services in the day surgery unit?
(3) What is the effect of the programme on nurses' satisfaction with their preparation of children and families for day surgery?
(4) What are the nurses' views of the amount of routine instruction administered on the day of surgery before and after the pre-admission programme?

Setting

The Izaak Walton Killam Hospital is a 185-bed teaching hospital which provides ambulatory and in-patient care to children in the Canadian Maritime provinces. The day surgery unit cares for approximately 25 to 30 children per day who are admitted for minor surgical procedures. The unit is staffed by five nurses who perform a brief medical history and physical assessment on each child pre-operatively and assist the family to understand the numerous events associated with day surgery. Parents are assisted to understand how they can help their child at key points in the day surgery experience. After the child's return from the recovery room, the nurses provide children with the physical care they require until they are awake and well enough to leave, and help parents to understand their responsibilities for care of their child at home.

Sample selection

A total of 75 families comprised the study sample: 23 families in the programme group and 52 in the non-intervention group. All families anticipating day surgery within the following week and who were within the hospital's local telephone exchange received a call inviting them to attend the programme on the Saturday morning preceding their child's surgery. The programme group families were selected by convenience from families who attended the programme during the period of data collection. The non-intervention group families were selected by convenience from all other families who were present in the day surgery unit during data collection periods with a child aged 3 years or older. The children in the programme group ranged in age from 3 to 12 years (M = 5.4 years). Those in the non-intervention group ranged from 3 to 15 years (M = 6.8 years).

The programme

On five consecutive Saturday mornings, families whose child was scheduled for day surgery within the following week were invited to a 1-hour programme at the hospital to prepare children and families psychologically for surgery. The programme was developed and delivered by the nurses in the day surgery unit and the senior nurse manager responsible for the unit. Second-year university nursing students assisted in the delivery of the hospital play component of the programme.

On the day of the programme, families were introduced to the day surgery unit and viewed a slide presentation of a family's experience at each stage of day surgery. The family depicted in the presentation was an actual family, consisting of a five year old boy and his parents who were photographed with their permission during the child's admission to the unit several weeks before the initiation of the programme. The family had received no coaching or special preparation for surgery and represented a coping rather than a mastery model. Then families were introduced to the pre-operative assessment procedures at which time the children rehearsed having their temperature taken electronically, tried on hospital clothes, and rehearsed weight, pulse and blood pressure taking. Reluctant children were encouraged to observe but not pressured to participate.

Children and families were then guided to the operating area where a nurse displayed her 'greens', mask, and boots and the children rehearsed saying 'goodbye' to their parents at the operating room door. Families then visited the recovery room and the children were reminded that they would be reunited with their parent when they awoke after surgery. After the tour, children and families assembled in the day surgery waiting area. The nurse conducting the programme met with parents to review the management of the common side-effects of anaesthesia and surgery and to assist parents to anticipate and feel comfortable managing the child's need for care at home after surgery.

The nurse provided parents with a handout which reinforced the programme information as well as some suggestions and resources for further psychological preparation of the child at home. In the same room but in a separate group, the student nurses used dolls and hospital equipment to help the children rehearse for day surgery, clarify their understanding of events, and practise the hospital procedures they had learned.

The evaluation procedure

On the day of surgery, immediately prior to the child's discharge from the day surgery unit, the research assistant approached the families and briefly explained the purpose of the study and the level of involvement associated with their participation. Then she administered a semi-structured interview guide which assessed parent and child anxiety at three points in the hospitalization (on admission to the unit, in the operating room waiting area, and at time of discharge from the unit), and asked what sources of information the family had used to become acquainted with the day surgery experience, as well as demographic information about the family, and parent and child's experience with day surgery.

Child anxiety was measured using the FACES Scale (Bieri *et al.* 1990), a self-report measure composed of seven faces that were derived from children's drawings of facial expressions of anxiety. The faces depict a range of experience from 'no anxiety' (1) to 'the most anxiety possible' (7). The child was asked to point to the face that showed how he or she felt at each phase of the hospital experience. Parent anxiety was measured using a 7-cm visual analogue scale. Parents and children were offered the opportunity to participate in the evaluation or not and assured that their decision would not influence the level of care they received. No parents or child refused their permission.

Data analysis

Descriptive statistics were used to summarize demographic characteristics of the children and families, as well as anxiety levels of parents and children at each phase of the experience. Differences in levels of anxiety between children and parents in the programme and non-intervention groups were compared using Cramer's V measure of association. The same statistic was used to test the association between child anxiety and previous child and parental day surgery experience, and differences in parental anxiety by experience with day surgery.

Results

A total of 23 families attended the programme and comprised the programme group. This number represents approximately one-third (32.6%) of the families who received a telephone invitation. Of the families who were invited and did not attend, over one-third said that previous experience had adequately prepared them for the present day surgery.

Children and parents reported similar patterns of anxiety in response to a hospital admission for day surgery. The highest levels of anxiety for both groups occurred in the operating-room corridor just prior to surgery. The children reported a mean anxiety score on admission of 1.69 (SD = 1.27). Those levels rose to 2.44 (SD = 1.88) in the operating-room corridor and decreased to 1.69 (SD = 1.39) prior to discharge. Parents also reported highest anxiety levels just before surgery (M = 2.77, SD = 1.89), followed by scores reported on admission (M = 2.03, SD = 1.72). Parents reported the lowest scores as they prepared to leave the hospital (M = 1.44, SD = 1.39).

Few children or parents reported anxiety scores of more than 4 at any time during the hospital stay. Therefore, in comparing anxiety scores the response categories of 4–7 were collapsed into a single category and the data were recoded according to four categories of anxiety instead of the original seven. An examination of the children's scores immediately prior to surgery revealed significantly fewer highly anxious children amongst those who had received the programme (Cramer's V = 0.33, $P \leqslant 0.04$) (Fig. 8.1).

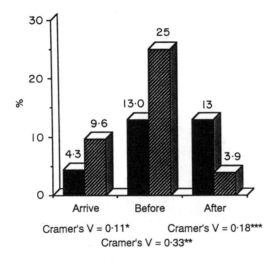

Fig. 8.1 Percentage of high child anxiety. Programme group ($n = 23$), ■. Non-intervention group ($n = 52$), ▨. *$P \leqslant 0.80$, **$P \leqslant 0.04$, ***$P \leqslant 0.49$.

Thirteen per cent of the programme group children reported high anxiety before surgery compared with 25% of the non-intervention group. This large difference was not observed at either of the other two reporting times. Parents in the non-intervention group consistently reported higher anxiety at all three times than those in the programme group but the differences were not significant (Fig. 8.2). A relatively strong and positive association was demonstrated between total child and parent anxiety (Cramer's V = 0.34, $P \leqslant 0.004$).

When non-intervention-group families described how they acquired information about day surgery, they identified the surgeon and the day surgery nurse as primary sources of information. Families rated the day surgery nurse higher than the physician, however, in their estimate of satisfaction with the information they received (Fig. 8.3).

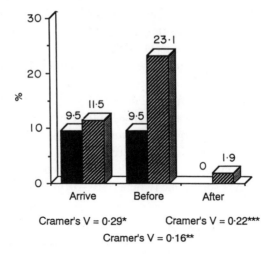

Fig. 8.2 Percentage of high parental anxiety. Programme group ($n = 23$), ■. Non-intervention group ($n = 52$), ▨. *$P \leqslant 0.10$, **$P \leqslant 0.56$, ***$P < 0.31$.

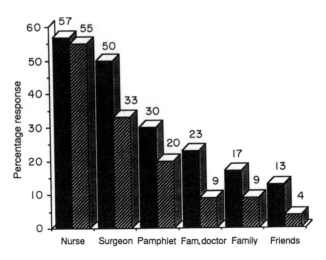

Fig. 8.3 Parent ratings of source and usefulness of information about day surgery ($n = 75$). Source of information, ■. Usefulness, ▨.

The responses from the programme group parents about the merits of the programme were positive. Of the 23 parents who attended, only two reported that they were less than very satisfied overall. Over 80% of parents rated the information component of the programme as very helpful for both parents and children. Somewhat fewer parents (74%) rated the programme as 'very helpful' in making the child or the parent more comfortable about the experience.

More than 40% of the parents and almost one-third of the children had previous day surgery experience. Children whose parents were attending day surgery for the first time did not report more anxiety on arrival at the hospital than those whose parents had previous experience. However, just prior to surgery, the rate of high anxiety was higher for children of experienced parents (Cramer's $V = 0.37$, $P \leqslant 0.05$); 35% versus 16% for the children of the inexperienced parents. There were no differences in the level of the children's anxiety at time of discharge from the unit regardless of parental experience. Similarly, almost twice as many children who had previous day surgery experience themselves reported high levels of anxiety just prior to surgery (Cramer's $V = 0.35$, $P \leqslant 0.08$); 33% of the experienced children versus 18% of the inexperienced ones. As well, more parents who had experienced previous day surgery with a child reported high levels of anxiety in the immediate pre-operative period (Cramer's $V = 0.40$, $P \leqslant 0.02$).

Preparation of families

The major incentive for the development of the programme had been the nurses' general observation that most families were not well prepared for day surgery. Nurses reported that often families came to the hospital frightened and without accurate information about the events their child would experience and how they could provide comfort and physical care for their child. The nurses anticipated that a programme would allow them to be more responsive to the individual needs of children and families for information and support and to achieve more personal satisfaction in their work. Overall, though, the nurses rated their satisfaction with their work relatively high: on a scale of 1 to 10, four of the five nurses related their satisfaction as 7 and one as 6. The nurses were interviewed again at the completion of the project. This time, four nurses rated their satisfaction with their work as 9 and one nurse as 10.

Three of the nurses reported that parents who had the tour were better able to help their children manage their anxiety on the day of surgery. They also reported that families who attended the programme retained information more easily than those who had not. For instance, one of the major problems the nurses described was the tendency for families to forget to ensure that their child fasted on the morning of surgery. None of the families who had the programme presented with this problem. The nurse also described a better rapport with families they met at the programme than with families who were new to them.

Discussion

Few children or parents reported very high levels of anxiety on arrival at the hospital, whether or not they had participated in the pre-admission programme. However, in the period just before surgery, more parents and children in both groups reported moderate and high anxiety than at the time of arrival at the hospital. One reason for higher anxiety just prior to surgery may be that the admission process is one which fully engages the family with activities. On the other hand, families wait as long as a half hour in the operating-room corridor without any responsibilities and with more time for reflection. The flow of patients and hospital staff through the operating room doors is a constant reminder of the imminence of the child's surgery. Several parents reported spontaneously that the most difficult part of the day for the parent and child was the point at which they were separated outside the operating room just before surgery.

There were few differences in reported anxiety between the programme and non-intervention groups. One explanation may be the self-selection of families of anxious children into the programme group. During most of the tours, at least one child was remarkable to the nurses for the child's demonstrated anxiety during the programme. For instance, one mother in the programme group initiated contact with the hospital herself for information about preparation because her two children were highly anxious about their upcoming surgery. The children appeared anxious during the programme, avoided eye contact with the programme activities and participants and refused to interact with the materials until the other children had finished playing with them.

One-third of the non-intervention-group parents who said they would not attend a programme if it was available had previous day surgery experience and felt that experience was an adequate preparation for this hospitalization. The fact that experienced parents and children reported higher levels of anxiety prior to surgery than those who were new to day surgery suggests that experience is not necessarily a good teacher and that recruitment efforts should target families with paediatric surgical experience.

Focus

The programme focused largely on familiarizing families with the sensations and the physical and procedural components of day surgery. Perhaps an extension of programme emphasis to include coping strategies for children and parents and opportunities to resolve concerns associated with previous hospital experiences may be effective in helping the families manage stress, especially stress associated with the waiting period in the operating-room corridor. The promotion of the programme to the physicians who use the day surgery service may also be helpful in encouraging more families, including those with experience, to take advantage of the programme.

The fact that the day surgery nurse was the primary source of helpful information to families suggests the limited preparation that most families bring with them to day surgery. However, the demands of a busy operating-room schedule leave the nurses little time for extensive teaching and psychological support in the hour before surgery. Receptivity to teaching is not high in this period either and supports the institution of a preparation programme which addresses the information and support needs of parents and is developmentally appropriate for their children.

The response by almost 40% of non-intervention-group families that distances from home would prevent them from attending a preparation programme is consistent with the hospital's records of rates of out-of-town patients. Most of those interviewed responded that they would have attended a programme if one had been accessible to them. A subsequent phase of this work included the development of an alternative programme of video and print materials suitable for families who cannot attend the hospital-based programme. That programme is now available to families through the provincial library system.

The large majority (74%) of children who attended the programme were of pre-school or primary-school age. The literature suggests, however, that school-age children also experience anxiety and are distressed by hospital experiences. Our experience with the older children who attended our programme supports that observation A programme that is targeted to older school-aged children and that acknowledges the information and support needs specific to this age group might be an incentive to school-aged children to participate in a preparation programme. In this study, families of children under 3 years of age were excluded from the programme because it was anticipated that very young children would not benefit psychologically from the experience. The fact that, overall, parent and child anxiety was moderately associated suggests that very young children and their families might benefit from parental participation in the programme even without the child's attendance.

Limitations

The retrospective reporting of anxiety was one of the limitations of the study. We felt it was too intrusive to approach families at three separate times during a stressful short-stay hospitalization for timely reporting of anxiety levels. Behavioural observations of children's and parents' anxiety by trained research assistants at the recording intervals might have provided more reliability for the self-reported measure of distress.

Conclusion

The study revealed mild to moderate levels of anxiety in children and families in day surgery. Anxiety peaked in parents and children just prior to surgery.

Attendance at the preparation programme was associated with lower levels of anxiety in both parents and children. That association was strongest in the period immediately before the child's surgery. Parent and child anxiety during day surgery were associated with previous surgical experiences.

The number and complexity of surgeries performed in day surgery continues to rise. Increased demands on the day surgery unit to accommodate more patients and the perceived importance of the nurse as a source of information and support suggest the value of the programme for families, especially those who anticipate difficulty in managing the stress associated with a day surgery experience.

References

Abbott, K. (1990) Therapeutic use of play in the psychological preparation of preschool children undergoing cardiac surgery. *Comprehensive Pediatric Nursing*, **13**, 265–77.

Ahmadi, K.S. (1985) The experience of being hospitalized: stress, social support and satisfaction. *International Journal of Nursing Studies*, **22**, 137–48.

Bieri, D., Reeve, R.A., Champion, G.D., Addecoat, L. & Ziegler, J.B. (1990) The Bieri pain scale. *Australian Journal of Paediatrics*, **16**, 23–30.

Johnson, J.E., Kirchoff, K.T. & Endress, M.P. (1975) Altering children's stress behaviour during orthopedic cast removal. *Nursing Research*, **24**, 404–10.

Lynch, M. (1994) Preparing children for day surgery. *Children's Health Care*, **23**, 75–85.

Melamed, B.G. & Siegel, L.J. (1975) Reduction of anxiety in children facing hospitalization and surgery by use of filmed modelling. *Journal of Consulting and Clinical Psychology*, **43**, 511–21.

Meng, A.L. (1980) Parents' and children's behaviour toward impending hospitalization for surgery. *Maternal–Child Nursing Journal*, **9**, 83–90.

Meng, A.L. & Zastowny, T. (1982) Preparation for hospitalization: a stress inoculation training program for parents. *Maternal–Child Nursing Journal*, **11**, 87–94.

Patterson, K.L. & Ware, L.L. (1988) Coping skills for children undergoing painful medical procedures. *Issues in Comprehensive Pediatric Nursing*, **1**, 113–43.

Roberts, M.C., Wurtle, S.K., Boone, R., Ginther, L.J. & Elkins, P.D. (1981) Reduction of medical fears by use of modelling; a preventive application in a general population of children. *Journal of Pediatric Psychology*, **6**, 293–300.

Sides, J.P. (1977) Emotional responses of children to physical illness and hospitalization. Unpublished doctoral dissertation, Auburn University.

Stewart, E.J., Algren, C. & Arnold, S. (1994) Preparing children for a surgical experience. *Today's O.R. Nurse*, **16**, 9–14.

Thompson, R. (1985) *Psychosocial Research on Paediatric Hospitalization and Health Care: A Review of the Literature*. Charles C. Thomas, Springfield, Illinois.

Vernon, D.T., Schulman, J.L. & Foley, J.M. (1966) Changes in children's behaviour after hospitalization. *American Journal of Diseases of Children*, **11**, 581–93.

Chapter 9
Analysed interaction in a children's oncology clinic: the child's view and parents' opinion of the effect of medical encounters

CHRISTINE E. INMAN, *MA, RSCN, RCNT*

Head of Nursing Development, School of Health and Social Welfare, Open University, Milton Keynes, England

Every effort is made to provide children affected by cancer-related illness with advanced medical care. This theory-developing, hypotheses-generating study focused on the child's view of the service provided in an oncology clinic. The methodology included interviews, observations of medical consultations and children's drawings. It also sought the parents' opinion of the effect of an impending appointment on the child's behaviour. The population for this ideographic research consisted of a convenience sample of 10 children over the age of 5 years, attending an oncology clinic which served a medium-sized city and its surrounding area. Quantitative and qualitative data were collected from semi-structured interviews, participant observations, transcribed audio-tape recordings and gaze interaction charts. Data were analysed using grounded theory. The medical interview was not acknowledge as being very significant by the children: their conscious attention centred on peers and play activities. The data also suggest that clinic visits are more acceptable for children when staff invest personal attention, give appropriate adequate explanations and handle children sensitively. Behaviour changes before appointments were reported by parents to be more prevalent in children who received less positive regard from the health team. Clinic observations and transcripts demonstrated the doctor's 'dominant role' during consultations. Interaction with the child centred around the examination and was frequently interrupted. A more extensive study would confirm or refute these provisional findings.

Factors which influence communications

Communication in a medical setting is complex because of influential interpersonal factors. In a paediatric oncology clinic, the complexity is increased by the number of people present, the uncertainty of outcome and the protective role adopted by the child's guardian.

Instead of dyadic patient–doctor interaction as in an adult consultation, the children's clinic can frequently involve the consultant, a medical register, a nurse, one or two parents, the patient and possibly siblings. These people all adopt specific roles to cope with the situation. Little has been written about the separate role of the child in a medical interview. In most instances the parent represents and replaces the child. The child is only required for the medical examination.

Parsons (1951) wrote extensively about the doctor and patient role. According to Parsons, the doctor is 'medically dominant' because of his 'specialised knowledge' and this creates a submissive, dependent patient. Despite this, the 'sick role' is described as being 'reciprocal and stable' because the participants have 'shared expectations'.

Bloor & Horabin (1975) doubted whether doctor and patient expectations were always shared and suggested that while many people accept the patient role, they may reject the 'sick role'. For paediatric oncology patients the sick role is avoided whenever possible to facilitate 'normalization' (Deatrick *et al.* 1988) or the maintenance of normal social and educational contacts.

Freidson (1975) questions Parson's (1951) view of 'medical dominance', suggesting that patients who are familiar with health topics may attempt to control the consultation. Doctors guard against such events because well-informed patients threaten their professional status. West (1976) states that knowledgeable parents of chronically sick children create 'dynamic interaction' with doctors. This also challenges the physician's authority.

Regarding making decisions, Waissman (1990) writing about a French population described decision-making as consisting of 'negotiation and conflict'. While the physician influenced the decision regarding the appropriateness of the home or hospital for the child's treatment, the final decision made by the parent could over-rule the physician's performance.

Strong (1979) is one of the few writers to consider the role of the child involved in medical encounters. Utilizing 'symbolic interactionism', he described 'role formats' in medical settings. These 'formats' were scarcely affected by the presence of the child. On the rare occasions when the child was invited to participate in medical interaction, the ensuing conversation was brief and could be interrupted by the parent. The child was treated as 'amusing, wonderful and innocent' but 'incompetent'.

More recently Waissman (1990) studied children requiring renal dialysis and found that the medical establishment and family could cooperate to the extent 'that the two parties could be said to form a single "family" for the ill child'. This also, by implication, suggests that the child could be excluded.

An unusual approach was adopted by Stimson & Webb (1975). They not only considered the child but actively sought his or her interpretation of a medical encounter. One hundred and fifty-one schoolchildren were asked to write an essay relating to a visit to the doctor. This revealed that on average 55% of essays were devoted to the period before the consultation, while only 36% were concerned with the actual medical encounter.

The child's involvement

The extent of a child's involvement in a medical consultation depends on age and maturity. Children can often converse with adults dyadically but have not acquired the technique to cope in complex polyadic situations (Forrester 1986). Another barrier relates to the use of gaze. Adults are accomplished 'multiple recipients' in group conversation involving gaze. Once again, children may not have learned these methods of gaining and retaining attention (Goodwin 1981). Yet another hurdle in group interaction is 'turn taking' in conversation. Children may attempt to become involved but their success depends not only on their skill, age and attention capacity, but also on the sensitivity of the adults present (Harrigan & Steffan 1983). Although young children may be excluded from adult conversation, recent studies indicate that they are 'skilful listeners', particularly when it comes to the 'process of overhearing' (Kraut *et al.* 1982).

Whether the interaction occurring during a medical interview is with the parent or child, there are many factors which influence it. When considering information provided for chronic patients, such patients are told more, more often and may even be given a better prognosis than people who attend less frequently, probably because their regular visits foster improved doctor–patient relationships (Joyce *et al.* 1976). Fletcher (1979) reinforced this point by noting that feedback is necessary for effective communication. Byrne & Long (1976) analysed feedback and discovered that doctors frequently 'listen selectively'.

Silverman (1987) carried this theme one stage further and produced evidence of parents also being given 'selective information' to obtain consent for investigations and treatment. The doctor does not deliberately intend to mislead the family but assumes that they are familiar with the procedure or technical language used, which inhibits understanding. Also relating to technical language, Korsch & Negrete (1972) noted that it produced monosyllabic responses from parents. Cartwright (1985) suggested that the 'social divide' and 'language problems' constrain working-class patients and can reduce interaction. In addition, parents found health professionals difficult to approach because they appeared 'busy'. Furthermore, parents feared a negative response to questions (Skipper & Leonard 1986).

Other forces which affect interaction

Non-verbal behaviour is known to affect interaction too. Heath (1986) noted the use of gaze to indicate whether the patient was receiving the doctor's full attention. Spatial arrangement, body posture and chair and desk position are also known to affect interaction (Matthews 1983).

Byrne & Long (1976) analysed speech during medical interviews. They discovered that a doctor influences the patient's readiness to interact by the type of questions asked. These can be 'broad openings', which encourage the patient to speak freely, open-ended questions which require a more limited response, and closed questions which need only 'yes' or 'no' in reply. They also described many other verbal influences on medical interaction.

In relation to the difficult task of communicating with adult patients with life-threatening conditions, the medical profession adopt an inconsistent approach. In a 1981 study, Gould & Toghill found that only nine out of 26 adult oncology patients were informed of their diagnosis early in the illness. Ideally, each family should be 'assessed individually' to discover their need for information.

The approach in paediatrics is usually more systematic. Shortly after diagnosis, young patients are informed in an appropriate manner of their condition, treatment and the side-effects. This avoids exposure to distorted versions via the playground or 'fellow patients' (Voûte *et al.* 1986). The effect of informing young patients of their condition varied with their age and sex. Older boys demonstrated a more realistic awareness than girls, while younger boys were more likely to develop psychological problems (Goggins *et al.* 1976).

The parents' ability to cope improved when they were given a totally honest account of the situation (Lascari & Stehbens 1973). Parents who were not given adequate information initially, expressed dissatisfaction. This complaint was particularly vociferous when the child was treated in two different hospitals (Peck 1979). Families appreciate almost any communication with the health team. Gould & Toghill (1981) divulged that even social chats with a doctor provided comfort and reassurance. 'Therapeutic interviews' which facilitated free talking by parents of children with leukaemia were also beneficial (Lewis 1967).

Suffering from a disorder with an unpredictable outcome influences interaction in a medical situation and affects patient compliance. Sociologists suggest that the extent to which doctors manipulate uncertainty affects their influence on the family (Waitzkin 1985; Stimson & Webb 1975; Carmaroff & Maguire 1981). In a review of childhood leukaemia, some children readily complied with therapy while others rebelled against their parents (Shapiro 1983). Adolescent patients who were conversant with their diagnosis and uncertain future were more likely to co-operate with treatment (Gould & Toghill 1981).

Anxiety

A British study of children measured uncertainty and anxiety during venipuncture. A clear correlation was demonstrated between adequate preparation with appropriate information and co-operation during the procedure and reduced anxiety (Rodin 1982). Jolly (1981) reinforces this view and suggests that some well-prepared children absorb sufficient knowledge to become 'mini-experts'.

We need, however, to consider the 'emotional state' which will affect how effectively they learn and may prevent the learning which is intended to prepare them and reduce anxiety (Weare 1992).

From a psychological perspective, a child who is perpetually anxious may be adversely affected by the subsequent stress. Rutter (1985) suggests that most children can cope with one major stress without developing psychological problems, but if two stresses occur simultaneously this 'enormously increases the possibility that the child will show serious symptoms'. Emotional symptoms were discovered in 40% of children attending the oncology unit at the Hospital for Sick Children in London. Howard (1979) suggests that this figure could be enormously reduced if each child was treated more sensitively when subjected to traumatic procedures. Pot-Mees & Zeitlin (1980) found that all children who had undergone bone-marrow transplant displayed emotional, behavioural and developmental problems. In addition, their parents had a 75% chance of developing depression.

Summary of literature

The multidisciplinary approach utilized in this review of literature was necessary because of the complexity of communicating in a medical setting. The evidence presented suggests that satisfactory interaction and sensitive management reduces anxiety, stress and consequently psychological problems for parents and paediatric oncology patients. Communicating effectively with these children is a daunting task when the variables involved are considered. These include the child's age, sex, social, emotional and education background and the rapport which exists between the child, parents and health team.

Methodology

The sociological perspective adopted was that of symbolic interactionism which utilizes methods advocated by Mead of the Chicago School (Mead

1934). He and contemporaries followed an anthropological approach. Fieldwork included observations, interviews and listening (Burgess 1982).

The population for this ideographic research consisted of a convenience sample of 10 children over the age of 5 years attending an oncology clinic which served a medium-sized city and surrounding area. The study focuses on each child's view of the service provided. The parents' opinion of the effect of an impending appointment was also sought. In addition, consultations with two physicians were observed, recorded and analysed to ascertain whether a structure existed and to discover contrasting elements which might emerge when doctors interviewed children.

Once the central idea for the study was determined, consent had to be obtained. Initially, this involved gaining the approval of the two consultants who conducted the clinic, the research and medical ethical committee and the nursing managers. The two clinic doctors readily consented and eventually the other powerful 'gatekeepers', the research and medical ethical committee and the hospital managers, also acquiesced.

The final vital stage of access was to obtain permission from the families involved. A formal informed-consent form was constructed and all the families involved in the convenience sample were approached either while waiting for a clinic appointment or at home. During this initial interview, rapport was established with the parent and child, as advocated by Oakley (1981), in preparation for more extensive interviews which were to be conducted at a later stage.

The pilot study

A trial clinic observation study was organized in another town at a hospital clinic conducted by a different doctor. This proved to be valuable for calculating how frequently it was feasible to observe gaze direction, the family's response to an observer being present and for estimating the Gestalt of the interview. Working alongside an uninvolved paediatrician also provided the opportunity for appraisal of the agenda prepared for the parent's interview. This improved face validity and prevented 'naive assumptions' from being made (Devons & Gluckman 1982).

The design

The population for this ideographic research consisted of 10 affected children over the age of 5 years. Seven of the patients were receiving therapy; three others who had completed treatment were attending clinic for routine checks. They were included to facilitate comparison.

Each child was audio-tape recorded and observed during a clinic appointment. In the 24-hour period before their next appointment, the child and parents were interviewed separately, at home when possible. A second observed and recorded medical interview was conducted during the child's next out-patient appointment.

The method

This study can be divided into three main areas: the child's view of the clinic, the parent's opinion of the effect of an impending clinic appointment on their child's behaviour, and the clinic observations. To discover the child's view, a non-scheduled standardized interview was used (Richardson *et al.* 1970). This type of interview helps in obtaining rich, descriptive data to discover attitudes, feelings and behaviour patterns (Hoinville & Jowell 1978). Open-ended questions were couched in a 'hidden agenda', inviting views and opinions. In addition, most of the children produced a drawing relating to an important aspect of their visit to the hospital. So 'multiple strategies' were employed (Burgess 1982).

Three methods were used for collecting information during clinic consultations. First, an audio-tape recording was made and transcribed. Second, observations of the gaze direction of the child and doctor were recorded every 15 seconds. Third, brief ethnographic notes were kept relating to the activities occurring within the consulting room. When combined, these three methods amount to a form of 'between method triangulation' (Denzin 1970).

Data analysis

For the child and parent interviews 'middle-range, substantive grounded theory' was the method most suited (Glaser & Strauss 1967). This provides an ongoing process where material is compared, then categorized as it is gathered. When categories become saturated, new ones are formed and other under-utilized categories may be combined. As categories are found to be interrelated, hypotheses begin to emerge.

Materials collected during the clinics were both ethnographic and numerical. The ethnographic material was subject to the above analysis; the numerical material provided quantitative data which were presented in charts. The charts facilitated comparison between doctors' interviews of the same and different patients. Statistical analysis was considered but the variables present were too great and the total sample too few.

The child's interview

Out of 10 interviews with children, six occurred in the home. Because of parental preference and educational demands, the other four took place in hospital during the generous wait for the medical interview. Ideally, the interview was to occur without a parental presence but it was difficult to stipulate conditions when favours involving access to offspring were being granted. Only three of the 10 interviews were with an unaccompanied child. Despite this, most consisted of relaxed after-dinner interaction with minimal parental involvement (Table 9.1).

Table 9.1   The site of the child's interview, parental presence and relaxed chatter.

The ideal	Successful	Unsuccessful
Home interview	6	4
Unaccompanied child	3	7
Relaxed chatter	8	2

When solitary and accompanied interview material was analysed, the content demonstrated little difference except that solitary interviews were longer and incorporated more irrelevant material. Of the 10 interviews, eight succeeded in encouraging the young patients to relax and chatter. Two home interviews were less successful: one because the child was pyrexial and unwell; the other was with a timid child who had had a bone-marrow transplant, whose social interaction with peers was minimal.

The non-scheduled standardized interview was brief in content. It focused on the child's view of 'good' elements of a clinic visit. This positive strategy was employed to avoid encouraging criticism. The researcher did not want to disrupt the child's ability to cope with appointments. Before embarking on the schedule, time was spent gaining the child's confidence by encouraging chatter about friends, personal interests, the school and home. Consequently, interviews could be relatively long. The eight successful ones ranged from 15 minutes to 1 hour.

The child's view of the clinic

Most of the children could recall one 'good' event relating to the clinic visit. The comment of one patient, who had completed treatment, was 'there's not very much to enjoy'. Other comments included, 'I like it especially when Imogen and Oliver's there because they're both my age', 'Chasing and playing tig around the corridors', 'When you've had your blood done and that you can go in the playroom', 'When they're all younger children you've got no one to talk to, that's when you usually use the teacher', 'I like the whole trip', 'Just riding my bike' at lunch time before the appointment, 'I like doing things ... like riding in the lifts', 'I like travelling when it's sunny'. For children who were unable to recollect anything pleasant, nine suggestions were made. They were travelling to the hospital, walking through the car park, riding in the lifts, talking to the nurses, doctors, teacher, play therapist and other children, and using the play equipment.

The positive aspects recounted are summarized and categorized in Table 9.2. Some children mentioned more than one positive activity; consequently the total percentage exceeds 100. The indications from Table 9.2 tie in with the children's statements cited at the beginning of this section. However, the child's low acknowledgement of interaction with the doctor is noteworthy. Some reasons for this were suggested:

(1) Other attractions involve the child and distract them from the consultation.
(2) Unlike school, the child has the freedom to select any available activity.
(3) The child can spend three or four times as long waiting, compared with the length of consultation.
(4) The child consciously or sub-consciously avoided considering the encounter with the health team as 'good' because of the associated treatment.
(5) The interaction with the nursing and medical team was not appropriate for the child.

Table 9.2   Clinic activities enjoyed by children.

Activity	Percentage	Treatment state
Interacting with peers	60	Children on and off treatment
Access to play equipment, teachers and play therapist	60	Children on and off treatment
The journey from school via home to the hospital, including the lifts	50	Children on and off treatment
Communication with the clinic nurses and doctors	20	Children on treatment

These or a combination of these factors could produce the above findings.

Whatever the rationale, the evidence derived from the interview was reinforced by pictures drawn by the children. Each child was asked to draw a picture depicting an important aspect of a clinic visit. Parents were asked to refrain from making suggestions or assisting. Due to maturity and illness, only eight pictures were received. Four were of the lifts and waiting areas which were situated next to each other. Three drawn by boys depicted the car and ambulance parks and hospital building. One picture was divided into four scenes; these followed the sequence of events which occurred during a visit – arrival by car, the hospital lifts, waiting with the other children and the clinic showing the nurse and doctor, not the mother and child. Five of the pictures were drawn while waiting at the clinic; three were drawn from memory at home (Table 9.3).

The subjects in the pictures emphasized the child's reluctance to consider the medical interview as important or enjoyable. Instead, the child's overt attention focused on the waiting period and the wider environment of the clinic.

Table 9.3   The children's pictures.

Scene	Percentage	Sex	Treatment state
The lifts and waiting area	50	3 girls	On treatment
		1 boy	Off treatment
Car park, ambulance, downstairs lifts and hospital buildings	37.5	3 boys	Two children receiving, one not receiving treatment
Picture divided into four scenes: Three scenes depicting the main events from arrival until the consultation One scene showing the doctor and nurse	12.5	1 girl	Receiving treatment via central line

Interviewing the parents

All 10 of the parent interviews occurred the evening before or on the morning of the patients' second observed appointment. All were arranged at times convenient for parents; nine were at home and one in an empty work-place staffroom. All were tape-recorded and most lasted for between half to one hour. Six were with mothers alone, four were with both parents. In three of these, the mother adopted the dominant role; in the other one, the father supplied all the answers. Most of the interviews were relaxed; one was less so because the patient was present and unwell. The hidden agenda for the non-scheduled standardized interview revolved around changes observed in the child's behaviour before an appointment. These included appetite, taking medicine, attitude towards school, ability to concentrate, thumb sucking and nail biting, the desire for extra cuddles, changes in toilet habits and anything else the parents had noted. Although the schedule was not extensive parents were encouraged to speak freely and this tended to promote 'therapeutic talking' which revolved around many connected issues. When the parent interviews were analysed, three main categories emerged regarding their opinion of their child's attitude towards visits and any associated changes in behaviour (Table 9.4).

Table 9.4   The parent's opinion of the child's view of the clinic and its effect on the child.

Group	Attitude and behaviour	Percentage	Treatment state
A	Child looks forward to attending clinic: no behaviour change	20	Two children receiving treatment
B	Child did not mind a quick visit: minimal behaviour change	40	One receiving treatment, three treatment completed
C	Child liked certain aspects of attending the clinic: extensive behaviour change	40	Four children receiving treatment

The first column in Table 9.4 provides two linked categories, the second refers to the percentage of children and the third to their treatment state. The two children in group A received extra attention from most people inside and outside the consulting room. One was an attractive, sometimes chatty 5-year-old with a chromosomal abnormality and articulate academic parents. The other was an 11-year-old, said by her father to 'love going to hospital' and she did appear to enjoy certain aspects of visits, in a quiet dignified way. During her usually unaccompanied consultation, however, the responsibility of coping alone made her appear rather apprehensive. On one occasion she displayed a 'healthy' anxiety regarding the date of her next injection.

Three of the children in category B had completed their treatment regimes, and consequently the physical trauma associated with clinic visits had ceased. Nevertheless, a reluctance to attend was reported by their parents. Perhaps this was due to memories of previous treatment days or the fear of relapse. Conceivably, it was because they visited less frequently so were unlikely to meet friends. Possibly, it was a consequence of attending after school, so forfeiting the privilege of time off. The later afternoon appointments also prevented children from making contact with the play therapist and teacher because they had completed their daily duties. A combination of the above factors may have influenced the child's attitude towards attending the clinic.

The fourth patient in group B was severely immunocompromised, and hence was permitted very limited social interaction. Thus, the opportunity for peer group contact at clinic compensated for some of the disadvantages associated with attending.

The four patients in group C were all receiving treatment. While they enjoyed the social and play aspects of the clinic, all their parents reported significant behaviour changes before appointments. These children exhibited alterations in appetite, mood, toilet habit and/or sleep patterns. As one mother summarized it, 'everything happens on clinic day'. Her daughter had developed shaking attacks. Another spoke of her child as 'very, very drained when she comes away from the hospital, it's almost as though she gets mentally prepared for it'. All parents believed their children coped better if they attended school on the morning of an appointment.

One of the most significant factors which emerged from this section was the consistent association observed between attitude and behaviour. The two children in group A highlight the potential benefit this correlation can endow. For entirely different reasons, they received more of the health team's attention and the parents also reported an absence of behaviour changes before appointments.

The clinic environment

The clinic was situated at the entrance of a general paediatric ward in the district hospital of a medium size city in the UK. This venue was used because qualified nursing staff were available to organize the clinic and the clinic rooms were adequately supplied with essential emergency equipment which may be required during bone-marrow or lumbar punctures. In addition, if the children attending clinic needed to be admitted, the ward bed state and facilities were immediately accessible. The ward staff were also able to maintain contact and develop relationships with children waiting.

There were two clinic rooms available, affording the two consultants facilities for conducting separate interviews to increase the efficiency of the clinic. Occasionally, the doctors participated in joint consultation if a patient needed extra attention or the clinic was relatively quiet. The social worker was also present in a separate room for patients who required assistance.

Unlike many out-patient clinics in the UK, all the children who booked to attend kept their appointments unless they were ill, in which case they invariably telephoned for advice. If any changes occurred it tended to be extra families arriving without an appointment because they were anxious about their child's condition.

It was usual for patients receiving treatment to have a blood test on arrival to enable results to be ready for the doctors when the clinic commenced. This encouraged some families to arrive early. Some went away after the finger prick to return later but others could wait in excess of an hour before the doctors even arrived. One parent described the waiting period as directly proportional to the level of anxiety experienced. Families developed 'coping strategies' to help them during this period. Some visited the voluntary service café in another part of the hospital. One child always brought a large bottle of fizzy drink. This frequently remained untouched but her mother said it was necessary to maintain the child's equilibrium. Another child's lunch-time cycling seemed to contain therapeutic properties. Possibly other behaviour 'rituals' would have been detected if sought.

The waiting area was not ideal considering patients could be severely immunocompromised. It consisted of a large square area where corridors and lifts converged. More suitable facilities had been offered to parents but they preferred to wait within sight of the consulting room doors. The children attending the clinic were provided with an excellent range of toys. They were also encouraged to utilize the play and schoolrooms on the ward.

When the young patients and their families eventually gained access to the doctor, the 'format' for each consultation followed a regular pattern similar to that described by Strong (1979). Within the pattern certain elements remained unique for each family (Table 9.5).

Table 9.5   The clinic format (reproduced with permission from Strong (1979)).

Greetings
Patient health (enquiries and discussion)
Examination
Treatment (omitted for children who had stopped treatment)
Next appointment
Farewells

Twenty-one medical encounters were observed; 10 with one doctor, 11 with the other. Two interviews were joint consultations. In both, one doctor directed the interaction while the other adopted a secondary role by only making an occasional remark. Of the 10 families involved, seven were observed during two separate consultations, two were seen on three different occasions and one only once.

The clinic data

The material collected in the clinic was collated and formulated on two charts (Tables 9.6 and 9.7). These summarize the data from the transcribed audio-tape recordings, the ethnographic notes and the gaze charts. (The transcripts of the audio-tape recordings will form the basis of a separate paper.) Tables 9.6 and 9.7 help to demonstrate the interaction which occurred in the clinic. They provide numerical evidence of the contrasting elements which occurred during medical encounters and they are indispensable for correlating the ethnographic observations.

On each chart, information is compiled relating to events which occurred in the clinics. They demonstrate the differences in doctors' style and also facilitate contrast between doctors with the same and different patients. Variation caused by interruptions from staff, letter writing, unwell patients, treatment and doctor or patient leaving the room are all accounted for within the chart. Despite the number of variables, the logical format in Table 9.5 remained constant. At the top of each chart is the clinic doctor's pseudonym

Table 9.6 Doctor Kent.

Pt	Age (yr)	Sex	Treat	TCT	TIP	NR and pauses %	DS-A %	DS-P %	PS-D %	DG-P %	PG-D %	DG-NI %	PG-A %	DS-M %	MS-D %	Comments
Ann 1																
a	8			8 min 55 s	8 min 55 s	28	51	3.5E 7.5C	4	9.5E 36C	7C	33.5	64	35	31.5	Patient unwell
b				27 min 2 s	24 min 4 s	21.5	44	16C	9.5	18.5E 23C	1E 6C	46	78	15	18.5	Injection Dr out
c	8	F	T													
Brian 2																
a																
b	5	M	TC	11 min 12 s	11 min 12 s	20.5	45	3E 20C	15	36E 22C	4.5E 15C	25	72	11.5	10.5	First doctor
Carol 3																
a				11 min 40 s	7 min 40 s	34	47	6.5E 21.5C	24.5	18E 36C	21C	30.5	61	11	14.5	Patient out
b	11	F	T													
c				25 min 25 s	21 min 55 s	37	48	7E 10C	13.5	14.5C	22.5C	60.5	76	12	14	Injection Patient out
Debra 4																
a				14 min 6 s	6 min 22 s	65	47.5	2E 4C	5	4.5E 13C	11C	73.5	80	27	26.5	Letter to hospital
b	8	F	T													
Edgar 5																
a				10 min 23 s	10 min 23 s	41	53	2E 16C	1.5	25E 19.5C	11C	33	89	18	Father 24	
b	5	M	T													
Frank 6																
a				10 min 31 s	10 min 31 s	19	46	6E 10C	11	21E 29C	13C	18.5	87	20	M&F 26	Patient on mum's knee after exam.
b	8	M	TC	9 min 11 s	7 min 3 s	13	52.5	2.5E 12.5C	12	20E 36C	28C	20	68	33	M&F 27.5	Patient out

	Visit	Age	Sex	Treat	TCT	TIP	NR and pauses	PS-D	DG-P	PG-D	DG-NI	PG-A	DS-M	MS-D	Comments
Gill 7	a	5	F	T											
	b														
Helen 8	a	11	F	T	3 min 12 s	3 min 12 s	28	57	47	33	54E 36C	64E 36C	9	27	5 No accompanying adult; Incomplete interview
	b														
Imogen 9	a	6	F	T	9 min 15 s	9 min 15 s	18	48	4.5E 13.5C	8	51E 19C	27E 6C	24	67	Grand-mother 13; Dressing changed
	b														
James 10	a	17	M	TC	7	1.5	0.5	8	51E 19C				0.5	2	0.5 Second doctor

a, b, c: a = 1st visit, b = 2nd visit, c = 3rd visit.
Sex: M = male, F = female.
Treat or T = treatment; TC = treatment completed.
TCT = total consultation time, in minutes and seconds.
TIP = total interaction potential.
NR and pauses = non-related speech and pauses.
DS-A = doctor's speech to anyone.
DS-P = doctor's speech to patient, E = examination instructions, C = conversation.

PS-D = patient's speech to doctor.
DG-P = doctor's gaze to patient. E = examination, C = conversation.
PG-D = patient's gaze to doctor. E = examination, C = conversation.
DG-NI = doctor's gaze to notes or instruments.
PG-A = patient's gaze anywhere except to mother.
DS-M = doctor's speech to mother.
MS-D = mother's speech to doctor.
Comments: these explain who was out of the room and so the time difference between TCT and TIP, and also any other major details.

Table 9.7 Doctor Lewis.

Pt*	Age (yr)	Sex	Treat	TCT	TIP	NR and pauses %	DS-A %	DS-P %	PS-D %	DG-P %	PG-D %	DG-NI %	PG-A %	DS-M %	MS-D %	Comments
Ann 1																
a	8	F	T													
b				11 min 58 s	11 min 58 s	19	5	0.25	0.25	1		1		4.5	4	Only entered
c							46	6E 17C	11.5	13E 32C	21C	26	58	23	30	briefly
Brian 2																
a	5	M	TC	8 min 39 s	8 min 39 s	42	49	4E 5C	4					31	29	No gaze chart
b							6	1E	0.5	7E 0C				1	0.5	Second doctor
Carol 3																
a	11	F	T													
b				8 min 37 s	8 min 37 s	31	41	5E 15C	11.5	31E 21C	27.5C	38	52	15	12.5	
c																
Debra 4																
a	8	F	T	20 min 51 s	12 min 20 s	47	47	4E 12C	13	8E 6C	2E 17C	75	25	26	Father	Dr out on
b																21	5 occasions
Edgar 5																
a	5	M	T	7 min 29 s	7 min 29 s	19	56	15E 15C	3	26E 15C	7.5E 3.5C	33	78	15	13.5	First doctor
b																
Frank 6																
a	8	M	TC													
b																

		Age	Sex	Type													
Gill 7	a	5	F	T	23 min 0 s	18 min 48 s	29.5	41	2E 11.5C	4	13E 26C	11C	36	82	25	26	Patient left room
	b				14 min 46 s	14 min 46 s	27	43	1.5E 11.5C	3	13E 39C	4C	26	83	28	33	Patient unwell
Helen 8	a	11	F	T													
	b				16 min 51 s	16 min 51 s	49	57	38	28	15E 19C	31C	55	38	5	3	Mum arrived near end
Imogen 9	a	6	F	T													
	b				23 min 42 s	23 min 42 s	20.5	49	5E 24C	16	7E 20C	9E 33C	66.5	40	14	17	Dressing and injection into line
James 10	a	17	M	TC	14 min 28 s	14 min 28 s	27	42	3.5E 20C	20	15E 7C	3E 17C	72.5	59	11.5	13.5	

See Table 9.6 for key to abbreviations.

(Tables 9.6 and 9.7). The patient's pseudonyms are in the left-hand column. This is followed by their age, sex and treatment state.

The number of times each child was observed in clinic is indicated by the letters a, b and c. Thus patient 1 was observed during three appointments. At the second consultation, Dr Kent was interviewing but Dr Lewis interrupted and participated briefly. Consequently, 1b has figures recorded both in Tables 9.6 and 9.7. Conversely patient 10 was recorded on only one occasion but again both doctors were present.

In the fifth column, the abbreviation TCT refers to the total consultation time from patient entrance to exit. This can differ from total interaction period (TIP) which records the length of time the major participants, the doctor and child, were both present in the consulting room. When total consultation time and total interaction potential differ, this indicates that the family has been excluded from interaction for the difference in these two figures. For example for 7a in Table 9.7, TCT is 23 minutes whilst TIP is 18 minutes 48 seconds. The reason for the difference is apparent from the 'comments' column which explains that the patient was out of the room for a period of time.

The remaining columns were expressed as percentages of the total consultation time. Non-related speech and pauses (NR and pauses) refer to cumulative pauses and speech which was not directed towards the family in the consulting room. It is the percentage of the total interaction potential during which neither the parent nor child were interacting with the doctor. NR and pauses range from 13% to 65%, producing a median of 28. Doctors' speech to anyone (DS-A) demonstrates the dominant role of the doctor. In every interview, the consultant spoke more frequently than anyone else present; the percentage ranged from 41% to 57%.

The next two columns are closely related; doctor's speech to patient (DS-P) and patient's speech to doctor (PS-D). Doctor's speech to patient is subdivided into speech related to examination (E) and conversation (C). Examination consists of instructions such as 'breathe deeply' and 'look at the poster'. These do not usually merit replies other than monosyllabic grunts and compliance.

The number of times the doctor addressed the patient and the patient replied may appear to be unrelated. For example in 1b the DS-P is 16% while the patient replies only 9.5% of the time. This imbalance can be accounted for by also examining the columns detailing doctor's speech to mother (DS-M) and mother's speech to doctor (MS-D). In this particular instance, the mother's replies exceeded the doctor's speech to parent because she was replying on behalf of her unwell offspring. In 6a, the imbalance occurred due to a particularly garrulous mother who prevented her child from participating in interaction to his full potential.

The remaining columns relate to recordings of the gaze direction of the child and doctor taken at 15-second intervals; doctor's gaze to patient (DG-P) and patient's gaze to doctor (PG-D). They are percentages of the total interaction potential. For both the child and doctor they were divided into conversation (C) and examination (E). During conversation, Dr Kent (Table 9.6) watched the children intently. This appeared to make most of the children withdraw their gaze. In nine interviews, the doctor gazed more frequently at the children. For the remaining two gaze observations, one (8a) was equal, whereas, in the other (3c), the child was receiving treatment and watched the doctor anxiously during the procedure.

In contrast, Dr Lewis (Table 9.7) spent a greater proportion of the potential interaction time gazing at case notes – doctor's gaze to notes or instruments (DG-NI). This allowed the child to inspect the doctor. In nine interviews with gaze observations, five allowed the child time to watch the doctor more often. In the remainder, the doctor's observations exceeded those of the child.

The excess of watching observed with Dr Kent appeared to inhibit the children, while Dr Lewis' attention to case notes made the child less self-conscious. The doctor's gaze also influenced the patient's utilization of gazing at anything other than the doctor–patient's gaze anywhere except to mother (PG-A). The final comment column extends the awareness of variables which were present.

Discussion

Although this research involved only a small sample, it succeeded in its stated aim of generating hypotheses. The first of these relates to the child's acknowledged view of the clinic which emerged from interviews and drawings. In both, the children emphasized the interval before a consultation rather than representing the medical encounter. The positive attitude to waiting may not have emerged if contact with peers, access to play facilities, professional educationalists and familiar health workers had not been available. Stimson & Webb's (1975) analysis of school children's essays also demonstrated the tendency of the child to focus on events occurring before seeing the doctor.

The second hypothesis is associated with the attention the child elicited from adults during a clinic appointment and the parent's opinion of the effect of a forthcoming appointment on the child's behaviour before an appointment. The children in Group A received more positive attention from the clinic staff than any of the other young patients. These children were said by their parents to anticipate forthcoming clinic visits with enthusiasm and did not display any adverse behaviour changes before an appointment. This suggests that health workers caring for children need to develop a greater awareness of their influence on the child's attitude towards clinic visits. While strictly comparable studies are not available, these findings correspond broadly with those of Jolly (1981), Rodin (1982) and Howarth (1979) who advocated providing appropriate preparation and sensitive handling.

Data extracted from the gaze charts form the penultimate hypothesis. The gaze measurements indicate that excessive scrutiny by one of the doctors caused many of the children to look away, which consequently reduced their involvement in interaction. The incidence of the first doctor's gaze being directed towards the child always exceeded all of each child's speech acts. Conversely, children attending the second doctor who received relatively less frequent scrutiny were noted to be more involved in the interaction which occurred and, for several, the child's speech acts exceeded the gaze incidence of this doctor. This suggests that the overwatched child is more likely to become detached from the interaction. An increased understanding of the effect of gaze is required by people involved in caring for children to ensure that the attention provided is acceptable to the child.

Finally, the clinic transcripts referred to in Tables 9.6 and 9.7 produced evidence of the doctors' total speech acts falling within a range of 41–57%, with both doctors in all interviews. As the doctor is responsible for conducting the interview, it seems reasonable to suggest that adequate interaction occurred during the majority of interviews, with the doctor maintaining the dominant role. During these interviews, serious topics were considered and, in contrast, social events such as holidays and celebrations were also discussed. Interaction with children was rarely lengthy and was likely to be fragmented, absent minded or interrupted either by adults or the examination. This correlates loosely with Strong's (1979) observation of the child in clinic being treated as a 'social object'.

Conclusion

This study demonstrates the value of adopting several methods of data collection. The findings which relate to the child's view of the clinic, and the parent's opinion of the effect of appointments on the child, broadly correlate. Both suggest that appropriate positive attention from health workers reduce the child's apprehension of appointments. These findings were reinforced by the clinic observations which indicate that the child had an adverse reaction to excessive watching by the doctor, which could be interpreted as inappropriate attention. To improve the situation, doctors could foster a sensitive approach to make visits to clinic more acceptable for children. In addition, supporting health workers could ensure that they complemented this practice.

Further research with a larger population would establish whether these ideographic findings could be applied nomothetically. A larger study would also clarify the relationship between improved health team interaction with children and the child acknowledging a more favourable view of the clinic.

References

Bloor, M.J. & Horabin, G.W. (1975) Conflict and conflict resolution in doctor/patient inter-actions. In *A Sociology of Medical Practice* (eds C. Cox & A. Mead), pp. 271–84. Collier Macmillan, London.

Burgess, R.E. (1982) *Field Research: A Sourcebook and Field Manual.* George Allen and Unwin, London.

Byrne, P.S. & Long, B.E.L. (1976) *Doctors Talking to Patients.* HMSO, London.

Carmaroff, J. & Maguire, P. (1981) Ambiguity and the search of meaning: childhood leukaemia in a modern clinic context. *Social Science and Medicine*, **15B**, 115–23.

Cartwright, A. (1985) Cited in Waitzkin, H. Information giving in medical care. *Journal of Health and Social Behaviour*, **25**, 83.

Deatrick, J.A., Knafl, K.A. & Walsh, M. (1988) The process of parenting a child with a dis-ability: normalisation through accommodation. *Journal of Advanced Nursing*, **13**, 15–21.

Denzin, N. (1970) *The Research Act.* McGraw Hill, New York.

Devons, E. & Gluckman, M. (1982) Cited in *Field Research: A Sourcebook and Field Manual* (ed R.G. Burgess), pp. 19–22. George Allen and Unwin, London.

Fletcher, C.M. (1979) Cited in *The Doctor–Patient Relationship: A Study in General Practice* (eds F. Fitton & H.W.K. Acheson), pp. 6–7. DHSS/HMSO, London.

Forrester, M.A. (1986) Polyadic Language Processes and the Pre-School Child. Unpublished PhD thesis. Department of Psychology, University of Strathclyde, Glasgow.

Freidson, E. (1975) Dilemmas in the doctor/patient relationship. In *A Sociology of Medical Practice* (eds C. Cox & A. Mead), pp. 285–98. Collier-Macmillan, London.

Glaser, B.G. & Strauss, A.L. (1967) *The Discovery of Grounded Theory Strategies for Qualitative Research.* Aldine, Chicago.

Goggins, E.L., Lansky, S.B. & Hassanein, K. (1976) Psychological reactions of children with malignancies. *American Academy of Child Psychiatry Journal*, **15**(2), 314–25.

Goodwin, C. (1981) *Conversational Organisation; Interaction Between Speakers and Hearers.* Academic Press, London.

Gould, H. & Toghill, P.J. (1981) Communication in medicine: how should we talk about adult leukaemia to adult patients and their families? *British Medical Journal*, **282**, 210–12.

Harrigan, J.A. & Steffan, J.J. (1983) Gaze as a turn exchange signal in group conversation. *British Journal of Social Psychology*, **22**, 167–8.

Heath, C. (1986) Participation in the medical consultation. *Sociology and Health and Illness*, **6**(3), 311–38.

Hoinville, G. & Jowell, R. (1978) *Survey Research Practice.* Heinemann, London.

Howarth, R. (1979) The child's response to the stress of a serious disease. In *Topics in Paediatrics 1: Haematology and Oncology* (ed R.H. Morris Jones). Pitman, London.

Jolly, J.D. (1981) Through a child's eyes: the problem of communicating with sick children. *Nursing*, **23**, 1012–14.

Joyce, C.R.B. *et al.* (1976) Cited in *Studies of Everyday Medical Life* (eds M. Wadsworth & D. Robinson), p. 4. Martin Robertson, London.

Korsch, B.M. & Negrete, V.F. (1972) Doctor–patient communication. *Scientific American Journal*, **227**(1), 66–76.

Kraut, R.E., Lewis, S.H. & Sweexey, L.W. (1982) Listener responsiveness and the co-operation of conversation. *Journal of Personality and Social Psychology*, **227**(1), 66–76.

Lascari, A.D. & Stehbens, J.A. (1973) A reaction of families to childhood leukaemia. *Clinical Paediatrics*, **12**(4), 210–14.

Lewis, I.C. (1967) Leukaemia in childhood: its effects on the family. *Australian Paediatric Journal*, **3**, 244–7.

Matthews, J.J. (1983) The communication process in the clinical setting. *Social Science and Medicine*, **17**(18), 1371–8.

Mead, G. (1934) *Mind, Self and Society: From the Standpoint of a Social Behaviourist.* University of Chicago Press, Chicago.

Oakley, A. (1981) Interviewing women: a contradiction in terms. In *Doing Feminist Research* (ed H. Roberts), pp. 30–61. Routledge & Kegan Paul, London.

Parsons, T. (1951) *The Social System*, pp. 428–73. Free Press, Chicago.

Peck, B. (1979) Effects of childhood cancer on long term survivors and their families. *British Medical Journal*, **1**, 1327–9.

Pot-Mees, C. & Zeitlin, H. (1980) Psychological aspects of bone marrow transplantations (BMT) in children. *Proceedings of the American Society of Clinical Oncology*, **4**, Abstract C. 984.

Richardson, S.A., Dohrenwend, B.S. & Kleine, D. (1970) Cited in *The Research Act* (ed N. Denzin), p. 125. Aldine, Chicago.

Rodin, J. (1982) In *Nursing Research: Ten Studies in Nursing Care*, vol. 2 (ed. J. Wilson-Barnett), pp. 157–77. J. Wiley & Sons, Chichester.

Rutter, M. (1985) Cited in *The Development Child* (ed H. Bee), p. 504. Harper Row, London.

Shapiro, J. (1983) Family reactions and coping strategies in response to the physically ill or handicapped child; a review. *Social Science and Medicine*, **17**(15), 913–31.

Silverman, D. (1987) *Communication and Medical Practice.* Sage, Bristol.

Skipper, J.K. & Leonard, R.C. (1986) Children, stress and hospitalisation: a field experiment. *Journal of Social Behaviour*, **9**, 275–87.

Stimson, G. & Webb, B. (1975) *Going to See the Doctor.* Routledge & Kegan Paul, London.

Strong, P.M. (1979) *The Ceremonial Order of the Clinic.* Routledge & Kegan Paul, London.

Voûte, P.A., Barrett, A., Bloom, H.J.G., Lemerle, J. & Neidhardt, M.K. (1986) *Cancer in Children.* Springer-Verlag, New York.

Waissman, R. (1990) An analysis of doctor–patient interaction in the case of paediatric renal failure: the choice of home dialysis. *Sociology of Health and Illness*, **12**(4), 433–51.

Waitzkin, H. (1985) Information giving in medical care. *Journal of Health and Social Behaviour*, **26**, 81–101.

Weare, K. (1992) The Contribution of Education to Health Promotion. In *Health Promotion, Disciplines and Diversity* (eds R. Bunton & G. Macdonald), pp. 67–74. Routledge, London.

West, P. (1976) The physician and management of childhood epilepsy. In *Studies in Everyday Medical Life* (eds. M. Wadsworth & D. Robinson), pp. 13–31. Martin Robertson, London.

Chapter 10
Factors influencing nurses' pain assessment and interventions in children

J.P.H. HAMERS, *RN, MSN*
Doctoral Candidate, Department of Nursing Science, University of Limburg, Maastricht, The Netherlands

H. HUIJER ABU-SAAD, *RN, PhD*
Professor, Department of Nursing Science, University of Limburg, Maastricht, The Netherlands

R.J.G. HALFENS, *PhD*
Associate Professor, Department of Nursing Science, University of Limburg, Maastricht, The Netherlands

and J.N.M. SCHUMACHER, *RN, MSN*
Inservice Educator, Spaarne Ziekenhuis, Heemstede, The Netherlands

Research is lacking on factors influencing nurses' decision-making directed at the diagnosis of pain in children and its related interventions. This chapter reports on two studies, a qualitative study and its replication, in which we explored factors influencing nurses' pain assessments and interventions in children. Those factors found to influence nurses' decisions were: medical diagnosis, child's expressions, age, and parents, and the nurses' knowledge, experience, attitude and workload. Some of these factors seem to have more influence than others. For example, the presence of a medical diagnosis seems to legitimate being in pain. Furthermore, it is suggested that mainly vocal expressions, especially crying, influence nurses' decisions to administer analgesics. Finally, nurses' negative views on non-narcotic analgesics were striking. The results of both studies and their relationship to information reported in the literature are further elaborated and discussed, and hypotheses on strength and direction of influence of factors on pain assessment and intervention are generated.

Introduction

In clinical practice professional nurses appear to make different judgements regarding the assessment of pain in children and the implementation of pain-relieving interventions. Assuming that it is desirable for nurses who are confronted with the same situation to make the same decisions, it is important to gain insight into the way decisions are made. A literature review conducted by the authors (Hamers *et al.* 1994) has shed some light on the subject and provided a framework of factors influencing the decision-making process. The literature review also reveals that most studies in nursing (Corcoran 1986; Tanner *et al.* 1987; Itano 1989) focus on differences in decision-making between the novice and the expert.

Research on other factors is lacking; for example, it is not known on the basis of which factors or cues nurses conclude that a child is in pain, or on the basis of which factors they implement interventions to relieve pain. Some authors (Broome & Slack 1990) stress that future research should be directed at answering questions such as: what criteria do nurses use to decide if a patient is in pain, and what factors do nurses consider when choosing medications to relieve pain?

The study

The purpose of this study is to explore factors influencing nurses' pain assessments and interventions in children. With this in mind, the research question was formulated: on the basis of what information do nurses assess acute pain in children, and what information do they consider when choosing pain-relieving interventions?

To answer the study question, a qualitative study was conducted (study 1) and followed by a replication study (study 2). In this chapter both studies, in which different researchers participated, are described.

Methods: study 1

Subjects

The subjects (*n* = 10) were a convenience sample of nurses (7 women and 3 men, average age 30 years) working on a paediatric ward in both a general and a university hospital in the southern part of The Netherlands. Seven nurses specialized in paediatrics; the other three had received training in this area. Experience in nursing varied between 1 and 14 years, experience in paediatrics between several months and 11 years.

Data collection and analysis

Date were collected using:

(1) Semi-structured interviews.
(2) Observations of subjects.
(3) Examination of nursing records.

The procedure was as follows: the main researcher joined the paediatric nurse during a daytime shift, observing the nurse's activities related to pain assessment and implementation of pain-relieving interventions. At the end of the shift, an interview with the nurse, recorded on audio-tape, took place. Owing to a technical malfunction, one interview was lost.

For data management the computer program KWALITAN 3.1 (Peters 1991) was used. KWALITAN has been developed for analysing data according to the grounded-theory approach (Wester 1991). By using KWALITAN the data can be processed, structured, sorted, selected, altered and printed. Furthermore, the program offers the ability to write, process and print (e.g. theoretical and methodological) memos. In short, the computer program offers the ability to apply the procedures for data analysis systematically on a large amount of data. However, it should be mentioned that it is not KWALITAN but the researcher who analyses and interprets the data.

During data analysis, memos were constantly written. Data were analysed using the following procedures. The main researcher and a second researcher independently coded the first interview. After comparing the codes, differences were discussed and agreement was obtained on terminology that should be used. The meaning of the codes was described in the memos. With these codes as a starting point, the main researcher coded a second interview. After the third interview was coded, no new codes could be formulated by the researcher, and the codes that were formulated seemed to be applicable to the different interviews.

At this time, procedures in data analysis were verified. First, both the content of the memos and the process of coding were discussed with the researcher who also coded the first interview. Next, they were checked by two other researchers, who assigned codes to randomly selected interview scenes. Results were tested using a similarity coefficient, the Jaccard index (see below). Based on the results of these measures, codes were readjusted. Data resulting from interviews, observations and nursing records were analysed on the basis of these codes.

Reliability and validity

In order to improve the reliability of data (Smaling 1987), interviews were tape recorded and transcribed. The computer program KWALITAN 3.1 was used in the data analysis. During the interviews the statements of the subjects were frequently summarized and restated by the main researcher. After doing the second interview, the interview technique was evaluated and discussed with three other researchers. During the data analysis, the main researcher regularly discussed methods and findings with colleagues, which supports reliability (Smaling 1987; Nievaard 1990).

To improve reliability and validity, the principle of triangulation (Denzin 1978; Kimchi *et al.* 1991) was also used. First, data triangulation was used by collecting data from a general and from a university hospital (dissimilar settings, Denzin 1978). Next, methodological triangulation was used by applying several methods of data collection: interview, observation, and analysis of nursing records (within-method triangulation, Denzin 1978). Finally, the research results were compared with the literature.

As mentioned earlier, the Jaccard index was used as a measure of similarity in coding between the main researcher and two other researchers (I and II). The procedure was as follows. Researchers I and II, neither of whom were trained in coding, had to code 10 randomly chosen interview scenes. They were given a list of 34 codes, each with a description of the meaning. They were allowed to use more than one code for a single interview scene, but not all codes had to be used. For every interview scene a Jaccard index could be calculated as a measure of similarity between two researchers (Table 10.1). According to Dormaar (1989), the Jaccard index is used in order to reduce the likelihood that two units would be considered similar because neither contains many of the attributes.

In this study, after readjustment of codes, the weighted similarity rates $[(J_1 + J_2 + \ldots + J_i/(n)]$ were: $J = 0.5$ (main researcher – researcher I), $J = 0.5$ (main researcher – researcher II) and $J = 0.4$ (researcher I – researcher II). These results have been interpreted to have reasonable similarity.

Table 10.1   The calculation of the Jaccard index according to Dormaar (1989).

The Jaccard, J, is calculated by the formula:

$$J = \frac{a}{a+b+c}$$

whereby a, b and c refer to the contingency table of attributes present (1) or absent (0):

	Researcher II	
Researcher I	(1)	(0)
(1)	a	b
(0)	c	(d)

Methods: study 2

Subjects

Study 2 was a replication of study 1. The subjects ($n = 10$) were a convenience sample of nurses (8 women and 2 men, average age 36 years) working on a paediatric ward in both a general and a university hospital in the western part of the Netherlands. All nurses were specialized in paediatrics. Experience in nursing varied between 5 and 33 years, experience in paediatrics between 2 and 28 years.

Because it was a replication of a study procedures and methods for data collection were the same as those described in study 1. As for reliability and validity, except for the use of the Jaccard index, those mentioned in study 1 were also applicable in the second study. There were, however, some differences, principally with respect to data analysis.

Data collection and analysis

Although the computer program KWALITAN 3.1 was used and memos were constantly written, data were collected and analysed by another researcher who did not participate in the first study. This researcher was trained in the interview techniques used in study 1. Moreover, to make the results of this study comparable to those of the first, the codes of the first study were used as a starting point in analysing the data. However, it should be noted that the researcher was not informed about the results of study 1.

Results: study 1

Factors found to influence both nurses' assessments of pain in children and the implementation of pain-relieving interventions are summarized in Fig. 10.1. These different factors will be discussed in succession.

Pain-relieving interventions can be divided into pharmacological and non-pharmacological interventions. Pharmacological interventions can be further divided into opioids/narcotics (e.g. morphine) and non-opioids/non-narcotics (e.g. paracetamol). However, in this report, when pharmacological interventions are mentioned they refer to non-narcotics.

Medical diagnosis

The medical diagnosis (surgery, syndrome, or indication for admission) is a factor that seems to influence nurses' pain assessments. Nurses seem to attach a great deal of importance to the medical diagnosis, since all 10 nurses

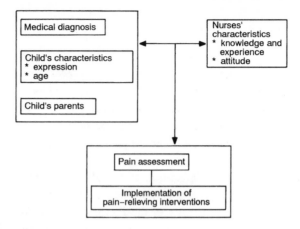

Fig. 10.1 Factors influencing nurses' pain assessments and interventions in children.

mentioned it. However, depending on the severity of the medical diagnosis, one may conclude that the more severe the diagnosis the more pain the patient experiences. As a nurse commented: 'The surgical removal of the tonsils [severe diagnosis] is more painful than the surgical removal of the adenoids [mild diagnosis]'. In fact, the presence of a medical diagnosis seems to justify being in pain.

> 'The assessment of pain also depends on the reason for the patient's admission to the hospital. A patient who is admitted with a medical diagnosis for which you can expect pain, is "allowed" to be in pain. It is to be expected.'

This observation also holds for the implementation of pain-relieving interventions. Medical diagnoses partly seem to justify the administration of analgesics.

> 'In the case of a child who has undergone surgery and complains about pain, there is a clear relationship between the operation and the reported pain. But when a child complains about pain as his parents are leaving, then distraction will be used [as an intervention].'

As in the assessment of pain, there is probably a relationship between the severity of the medical diagnosis and the nurse's decision, in this case the implementation of a pain-relieving intervention. One will be more inclined to administer an analgesic with a severe diagnosis than with a mild diagnosis.

Characteristics of the child

Certain characteristics of the child will influence nurses' pain assessments, mainly the child's expressions and the child's age.

The child's expressions

The child's expressions seem to be an important cue in pain assessment. Although there are many ways – vocal/verbal, facial, behavioural, body movements – in which a child can express pain, vocal and verbal expressions are those that influence the assessment the most. Crying seems to be the most reliable source. In other words, the likelihood that a child will be in pain increases if the child is crying. This conclusion is based on the large number of scenes in which respondents mention the importance of this cue.

All nurses state that a child can be asked if he is in pain and that children can and do report their pain verbally. However, nurses have their doubts about the reliability of this source of information:

'Older children can express this verbally. They say, "I have a stomach ache." Then you need to watch and see if that really is true or whether what they really mean to say is, "I want to go home." '

As with pain assessment, vocal and verbal expressions also seem to influence the implementation of pharmacological interventions. In other words, a shouting or crying child will receive a pain medication sooner than a child who is not reacting in such a verbal manner.

'When the child is lying in bed screaming in pain, there is not much point in trying to reposition him. You just reach for some medication.'

The child's age

With regard to age, respondents distinguish between 'younger children' (up to 4 years old), 'older children' (starting at 5 years old) and 'adults'. The majority of the subjects think of age as a factor that influences pain assessment. However, they do not agree on the nature of the influence. Some of the nurses think adults experience more pain than children in the same situation. Reasons given are:

'I think children forget it more quickly. An adult who has a hernia will stay in bed for about 2 days and take it easy, while a child will start walking around or playing within a couple of hours. He won't think about it that much.'

However, the majority of the nurses think children experience more pain than adults in the same situation. Several arguments are brought up, for instance:

'An adult may be able to handle it better than a child. When a child is in pain, he is totally overwhelmed by it. He can think of nothing else. He can't even play anymore.'

It is less clear whether nurses think that younger children have more or less pain than older children in the same situation. One subject stated:

'The conclusion that the child is in pain will be drawn more quickly for younger children than for older children. With the younger child you play it safe; with the older one you check it.'

Age also seems to influence the implementation of pharmacological interventions. Several nurses think adults receive pain medication sooner than children.

'Compared with children, adults receive medication more quickly.'

One nurse thinks the decision to administer an analgesic is made more quickly in younger children than in older children.

'In infants you tend to give something [analgesic] more quickly. If the child remains restless, then he is experiencing pain. This conclusion will be drawn earlier than in older children.'

The child's parents.

In general, subjects think it is obvious to use information obtained from the child's parents. After all, 'Nobody knows the child better than his own parents'. However, information obtained from parents does not seem to be reliable all the time. When a parent states that her child is in pain, this information is usually checked by the nurse.

'Parents do recognize the child's pain behaviour; it is specific for their child. Still, you first have to assess the situation yourself. If the child hears a parent say, "If I had undergone that operation I would have had pain", he will begin to experience pain himself.'

Other nurses check whether the pain is severe enough to administer pain medication.

'In that case I will go back with them [parents] to their child, and talk with the child himself [if that is possible]. That way, I can decide whether to administer pain medication or not.'

The reliability of the parent's information depends on the subject's image of the parents.

'Sometimes it's obvious that the parents are exaggerating.'

Characteristics of the nurse

Nurses appear to know that they make different decisions when confronted with the same situation. These differences can be partly attributed to nurses' characteristics, including their knowledge, experience and attitude.

Knowledge and experience

Professional experience seems to be a main factor influencing nurses' pain assessments and their implementation of interventions. Nurses use their past experience to determine what to do in present or future situations.

> 'Experience with the syndrome, experience with other children. You start making comparisons. Actually, I shouldn't be saying this, but is it logical to be in pain? You should bear in mind that every human being is unique. But the fact is you do it [comparing] automatically, you cannot avoid it.'

Knowledge about the effects of pain-relieving interventions seems to influence nurses' implementation of them. Analgesics are generally expected to be effective. That cannot be said of non-pharmacological interventions. The non-pharmacological intervention most often mentioned is distraction. Some nurses think distraction can be an effective way to relieve pain. Other nurses think distraction is a temporary solution, and not a sufficient one. Finally, other nurses think of distraction as a method of assessing, rather than relieving, pain.

> 'Distraction is a kind of test to assess the severity of pain.'

Nurses' attitudes

Nurses' attitudes seem quite likely to influence their decision to administer pain medication to children. It appears that nurses have negative feelings about pain medication, a conclusion derived from the vocabulary they use: 'All pain will be treated, if necessary even with medicines'; 'If I start stuffing them with medicine...'; 'Then you don't need to start pushing medicines right away'; 'You shouldn't pump it into the body if it is not necessary'; 'You don't need to swallow packets of pills'. These statements give the impression that the nurses are talking about large quantities of medicine. However, the context of these statements is the administration of 'paracetamol' prn. Moreover, it is striking that nurses postpone administering analgesics as long as possible.

> 'In my opinion it is not necessary to start with an analgesic right away. In fact, as far as that's concerned, I would say, wait until the last possible moment.'

Several arguments are given for postponing the administration of analgesics: 'because medicine is harmful'; 'because it is a poison'; 'because medicine has side-effects'; 'because medicine suppresses other symptoms'; 'because you are afraid something is going to go wrong'.

Finally, the majority of nurses think that pain is related to hospital admission. Some of them think that pain can never be relieved completely.

'In fact, some pain is allowed, for they are, after all, in hospital.'

Results: study 2

An extensive overview of the results of this replication study is given by Schumacher (1993). Obviously, in general, the results of this study were comparable to those of the first one. The impact of the medical diagnosis on assessment and intervention was supported. This also held for the child's expressions, nurses' knowledge and experience, and nurses' attitude.

However, there were some differences with regard to the influence of the child's age on the pain assessment and administration of analgesics. In study 1, it was suggested that younger children would probably receive pain medication earlier than older children. Study 2 suggests conflicting results. On the one hand, the result is supported.

'To older children, you can say, "Hang in there!" ... but this is not going to work with younger children.'

On the other hand, some subjects suggest the opposite; older children would receive pain medication earlier.

'In younger children pain is managed less extensively than in older children.
In younger children, you first try out other [non-pharmacological] interventions.'

Although the influence of the child's parents is supported, the examination of information from parents was not mentioned. However, the parent's influence on the nurse's decision to administer an analgesic seems rather small.

'You only have a few alternatives and the parents don't have much to say in the matter.'

Finally, an interesting result found in this study was the influence of 'workload' on the administration of analgesics.

'My first reaction is not very acceptable, but it depends on how much time you have available. When you are caring for 13 children all by yourself, or with another colleague, then you do not have enough time to sit down with each child.'
'When it is very busy, and you are caring for 12 children all by yourself, then you naturally just give a paracetamol.'

In such cases, time seems to be a determining factor in the administration of analgesics.

Discussion

Decision-making processes related to pain assessment and interventions in children are complicated. In a qualitative study, followed by a replication study, factors influencing these processes have been explored. It should be mentioned that the overview is not complete; for example, organizational aspects (Broome & Slack 1990) were left aside, although there was an indication that workload also influences the administration of analgesics (study 2). Obviously, the subjects do not represent all paediatric nurses in the Netherlands, something which sets limitations on the range of these studies. However, it does not alter the fact that clear indications have been found about the influence of some factors on nurses' decision-making.

Medical diagnosis

A medical diagnosis seems to be a justification for being in pain. The importance of the medical diagnosis in pain assessment and interventions has also been reported in the literature (Dudley & Holm 1984; Taylor *et al.* 1984; Burokas 1985; Arkesteyn 1989; Bush *et al.* 1989; Halfens *et al.* 1990; Ross *et al.* 1991). These findings lead one to believe that the worse the medical diagnosis, the higher the pain assessment and the sooner an analgesic will be administered.

Child's expressions

The finding that nurses use the child's expressions to assess pain seems logical. The overview of the ways in which a child can express pain is comparable to overviews which exist already (McGrath & Unruh 1987; Ferrell *et al.* 1991; Koolen & Perduijn 1991). However, it is striking that mainly vocal and verbal expressions, especially crying, influence nurses' decisions. This finding is contrary to results of two other qualitative studies which suggest that nurses assessing pain pay the most attention to the child's behaviour (e.g. reflecting boredom, introversion) (Koolen & Perduijn 1991) and facial expression (e.g. grimace, frown) (Dick 1993). Dick's study (1993) also suggests that crying may be an important cue. A study by Wallace (1989) again supports the finding that children who express pain intensively receive more postoperative analgesic medication than children who express pain less intensively.

Age

The influence of age on pain assessment and intervention is also worth noting. The majority of nurses believe that children have less pain than adults in the same situation. According to McGrath *et al.* (1984), there is no difference in perceived pain of children and adults when no serious medical sequela is expected. The finding that adults seem to receive analgesics sooner than children is supported in the literature (Eland & Anderson 1977; Beyer *et al.* 1983; Schechter *et al.* 1986; Elander & Hellström 1992).

The assumption that younger children, especially babies, do not feel pain seems to be obsolete. The present study even suggests that nurses conclude that younger children are in pain sooner than older children. A younger child is also likely to be given analgesics sooner. An explanation for this could be that it is more complicated to assess pain in younger children than in older children. As a result, nurses will administer analgesics sooner to be on the safe side. Moreover, it is assumed that pain assessment in older children is less complicated because they can report their pain verbally. Some nurses, on the other hand, still debate the reliability of these reports. A child who reports pain may be simulating or exaggerating pain, something that is also suggested in the literature (Koolen & Perduijn 1991; Vortherms *et al.* 1992).

Regarding the influence of age on the administration of analgesics, conflicting findings exist not only in study 2 but also in the literature. According to Elander & Hellström (1992), older children received more narcotic analgesics but got the same amount of non-narcotic analgesics as younger children. Gonzalez & Gadish (1990) suggest that younger children receive more non-narcotics than older children. However, nurses who participated in this study said that age is not an important factor in influencing the administration of analgesics. This idea is supported by Schechter *et al.* (1986). These researchers found that narcotic analgesics are prescribed less often in younger children than in older children, but that there is no difference in the actual administration.

In summary, different results have been reported regarding the influence of age on pain assessment and interventions. Therefore, it remains questionable whether age (younger versus older children) influences the decision to administer analgesics.

Influence of parents

It is also questionable whether a child's parents influence nurses' pain assessments and interventions. Although subjects think information obtained from parents is important, study 1 suggests that this information must be confirmed. In any case, information obtained from parents seems unlikely to be a conditional factor for the administration of analgesics. These findings are supported by those of Koolen & Perduijn (1991). These authors also support the finding that the parents' role is age-related. In other words, if information obtained from parents influences nurses' decision-making, this influence decreases as the child grows older. In the literature the child's parents as an influencing factor on nurses' decisions is seldom described.

Nurses' attitudes

It seems logical to conclude that nurses' characteristics influence their decisions. However, nurses' attitudes towards analgesics are striking. In the literature (Eland & Anderson 1977; Schechter *et al.* 1986; Ferrell *et al.* 1991) it is often mentioned that many nurses are (sometimes unjustly) afraid of side-effects of analgesics, like addiction. These studies, however, refer to narcotic analgesics, while the qualitative study and its replication reflect negative views on non-narcotic analgesics, like paracetamol. It is possible that children receive insufficient analgesics as a result of this, or that analgesics are administered too late.

Distraction

Distraction seems to be the non-pharmacological intervention most often used, a finding supported by Burokas (1985). However, it seems that the range of non-pharmacological interventions used is less than the range of non-pharmacological interventions described in the literature (Ross & Ross 1988; Huijer Abu-Saad 1989; McGrath 1990). This observation is also made by Ferrell *et al.* (1991). An explanation could be that few nurses are acquainted with non-pharmacological interventions and their effects. Moreover, it is likely that several interventions that are described in the literature (e.g. hypnosis and biofeedback) are not considered within the nursing domain in The Netherlands.

Implications for future research and clinical practice

Based on this study, several suggestions for further research can be made. The results of this study are hypothetical in nature. Testing hypotheses, particularly on the influence of medical diagnosis, the child's expressions and age, and the child's parents, should be the next step. Further research on nurses' attitude towards pain in children seems to be relevant, all the more so because nurses' attitudes seem to be responsible for differences between nurses' decisions to administer analgesics. Finally, one should investigate whether or not children receive sufficient analgesics.

This study also has practical implications, especially for nursing education and nursing practice. It is suggested that nurse educators should pay more attention to pain assessment and to methods of relieving pain in children, taking into consideration analgesics and their side-effects. In addition, the subjective nature of the experience and the developmental influences on pain perception, pain tolerance and pain expression in children should receive more attention in nursing school curricula.

In the practice setting, refresher courses on pain in children are recommended for paediatric nurses because they are the ones who determine if a child is to be medicated or not and because they are seen as role models by potential nursing students in the practical setting. Refresher courses could address how children with different medical diagnoses and of different age groups perceive and react to painful experiences. Myths regarding pain assessment and pain management in children could be discussed and as a result dispelled.

References

Arkesteyn, S.A.C. (1989) Onderzoek naar factoren die verpleegkundigen beïnvloeden bij het toedienen van postoperatieve pijnmedicatie bij kinderen. (Research on factors influencing nurses' administration of analgesics in children postoperatively.) Unpublished doctoral thesis. Rijksuniversiteit Limburg, Maastricht.

Beyer, J.E., DeGood, D.E., Ashley, L.C. & Russell, G.A. (1983) Patterns of postoperative analgesic use with adults and children following cardiac surgery. *Pain*, **17**, 71–81.

Broome, M.E. & Slack, J.F. (1990) Influence on nurses' management of pain in children. *Maternal Child Nursing*, **15**, 158–62.

Burokas, L. (1985) Factors affecting nurses' decisions to medicate pediatric patients after surgery. *Heart & Lung*, **14**(4), 373–9.

Bush, J.P., Holmbeck, G.N. & Cockrell (1989) Patterns of PRN analgesic drug administration in children following elective surgery. *Journal of Pediatric Psychology*, **14**, 433–48.

Corcoran, S.A. (1986) Task complexity and nursing expertise as factors in decision making. *Nursing Research*, **35**(2), 107–12.

Denzin, N.K. (1978) *The Research Act. A Theoretical Introduction to Sociological Methods.* McGraw-Hill, New York.

Dick, M.J. (1993) Preterm infants in pain. Nurses' and physicians perceptions. *Clinical Nursing Research*, **2**(2), 176–87.

Dormaar, J.M. (1989) *Consensus in Psychotherapy.* Datawyse, Maastricht.

Dudley, D.R. & Holm, K. (1984) Assessment of the pain experience in relation to selected nurse characteristics. *Pain*, **18**, 179–86.

Eland, J.M. & Anderson, J.E. (1977) The experience of pain in children. In *Pain: A Source Book for Nurses and Other Health Professionals* (ed. A. Jacox), pp. 453–73. Little, Brown, Boston.

Elander, G. & Hellström, G. (1992) Analgesic administration in children and adults following open heart surgery. *Scandinavian Journal of Caring Sciences*, **6**(1), 17–21.

Ferrell, B.R., Eberts, M.T., McCaffery, M. & Grant, M. (1991) Clinical decision making and pain. *Cancer Nursing*, **14**(6), 289–97.

Gonzalez, J. & Gadish, H. (1990) Nurses' decisions in medicating children postoperatively. In *Advances in Pain Research and Therapy* (eds D.C. Tyler & E.J. Krane), pp. 37–41. Raven, New York.

Halfens, R., Evers, G. & Abu-Saad, H. (1990) Determinants of pain assessment by nurses. *International Journal of Nursing Studies*, **27**(1), 43–9.

Hamers, J.P.H., Huijer Abu-Saad, H. & Halfens, R.J.G. (1994) The diagnostic process and decision-making in nursing, a literature review. *Journal of Professional Nursing*, **10**(3), 154–63.

Huijer Abu-Saad, H. (1989) Pijninterventies bij kinderen. (Pain interventions in children.) *Pijn-Informatorium*, **15**, 1–13.

Itano, J.K. (1989) A comparison of the clinical judgment process in experienced registered nurses and student nurses. *Journal of Nursing Education*, **28**(3), 120–26.

Kimchi, J., Polivka, B. & Stevenson, J.S. (1991) Triangulation: operational definitions. *Nursing Research*, **40**(6), 364–6.

Koolen, Y.H.E. & Perduijn, M.D. (1991) *Clinical Judgment. Acutely and Chronically Ill Children in Pain*. Unpublished doctoral thesis. Rijksuniversiteit Limburg, Maastricht.

McGrath, P.A. (1990) *Pain in Children, Nature, Assessment and Treatment*. Guildford, New York.

McGrath, P.J. & Unruh, A.M. (1987) *Pain in Children and Adolescents*. Elsevier, Amsterdam.

McGrath, P.J., Vair, C., McGrath, M.J., Unruh, E. & Schnurr, R. (1984) Pediatric nurses perception of pain experienced by children and adults. *Nursing Papers*, **16**, 34–40.

Nievaard, A.C. (1990) Validiteit en betrouwbaarheid in kwalitatief onderzoek. Validity and reliability in qualitative research.In *Objectiviteit inKwalitatief Onderzoek*. (Objectivity in qualitative research.) (eds I. Maso & A. Smaling). Boom, Meppel.

Peters, V. (1991) *Kwalitan, Aanvullende Handleiding bij Versie 3.1*. (Kwalitan, manual for version 3.1.) Katholieke Universiteit, Nijmegen.

Ross, D.M. & Ross, S.A. (1988) *Childhood Pain. Current Issues, Research, and Management*. Urban & Schwarzenberg, Baltimore.

Ross, R.S., Bush, J.P. & Crumette, B.D. (1991) Factors affecting nurses' decisions to administer PRN analgesic medication to children after surgery: an analog investigation. *Journal of Pediatric Psychology*, **16**(2), 151–67.

Schechter, N.L., Allen, D.A. & Hanson, K. (1986) Status of pediatric pain control: a comparison of hospital analgesic usage in children and adults. *Pediatrics*, **77**(1), 11–15.

Schumacher, J. (1993) *Verpleegkundige Besluitvorming: Pijn bij Kinderen*. (Decision-making in nursing: pain in children.) Unpublished doctoral thesis. Rijksuniversiteit Limburg, Maastricht.

Smaling, A. (1987) *Methodologische Objectiviteit en Kwalitatief Onderzoek*. (Methodological objectivity and qualitative research.) Swets & Zeitlinger, Lisse.

Tanner, C.A., Padrick, K.P., Westfall, U.A. & Putzier, D.J. (1987) Diagnostic reasoning strategies of nurses and nursing students. *Nursing Research*, **36**(6), 358–63.

Taylor, A.G., Skelton, J.A. & Butcher, J. (1984) Duration of pain condition and physical pathology as determinants of nurses' assessments of patients in pain. *Nursing Research*, **33**(1), 4–8.

Vortherms, R., Ryan, P. & Ward, S. (1992) Knowledge, attitudes toward, and barriers to pharmacologic management of cancer pain in a statewide random sample of nurses. *Research in Nursing and Health*, **15**, 459–66.

Wallace, M.R. (1989) Temperament: a variable in children's pain management. *Pediatric Nursing*, **15**(2), 118–21.

Wester, F. (1991) *Strategieën voor Kwalitatief Onderzoek* (Strategies for qualitative research.) Coutinho, Muiderberg.

Chapter 11
The changing role of the nurse in neonatal care: a study of current practice in England

ANNE HARRIS, *RN*

Research Associate, Department of Child Health, University of Bristol, Royal Hospital for Sick Children, Bristol, England

and MARGARET REDSHAW, *BA, PhD*

Research Fellow, Neonatal Nurses Project, Department of Child Health, University of Bristol, Royal Hospital for Sick Children, Bristol, England

The boundaries of nursing in neonatal care, and the interface between the work of nursing and medical staff in delivering care, are changing. The enhanced or expanding role of the neonatal nurse is not a universally accepted one. If this professional development is to be widely accepted and implemented, some key issues will need to be addressed so that the changing role of the nurse and associated skill base are well founded. As part of a large-scale national study of neonatal nursing in England, data were collected from nurses working in 24 different units. Regional centres, subregional centres and district units from six widely separated health regions participated, and individual data were collected from 718 nurses (599 D–I grades and 119 A–C grades). While indicating that there is inter-unit variation in nursing practice, the results also show that many nurses are already in the process of changing their role in this acute specialty. Nurses doing so are more likely to have a qualification in this specialty, though not all of them had such post-registration training. A small number of nursery nurses and nursing auxiliaries were undertaking tasks that could be considered part of an expanded role. The implications of the findings are discussed.

Introduction

During its evolution, the field of neonatology has seen rapid advances in terms of the knowledge and expertise needed to care for increasing numbers of small, sick newborn babies (Harvey *et al.* 1989; Audit Commission 1993; Roberton 1993). With this developing understanding and advances in technology, nursing and medical techniques have been refined. Nurses working in this area have developed a skill base from which to deliver both technical and practical care, and this is now embodied in the post-registration courses providing specific training in special and intensive care of the newborn.

Development of the nurse's role in neonatal care has taken place in a number of countries, commonly in response to medical staffing crises (Boxall 1987). In the United States, advancement of the role has largely taken place in a technical direction, encompassing a wide range of practical clinical procedures (Karp 1993). In Canada, although the role is clinically focused and contains a technical element, relatively greater emphasis has been placed on expanding the nursing role in areas that include administration, teaching, parental support, and research (Herbert & Little 1983; Beresford 1991).

Advanced nurse practitioner

Interest in the concept of the advanced nurse practitioner in the UK has recently been developing (Chiswick & Roberton 1987; Hale *et al.* 1987). Findings from a survey by the National Association of Neonatal Nurses on neonatal nurse practitioners concluded that, while it was important to look to the future, there were reservations about development of the role (Boxall 1987; Hall *et al.* 1992). Fundamental issues such as staffing adequacy, remuneration, career structure, and the goal of delivering holistic family care, will need to be addressed in addition to immediate training requirements.

Recent studies in the UK have focused on the role of the nurse in high-technology areas (Youngman *et al.* 1988; DoH 1989; Stock & Ball 1992), looking at qualifications in specialty, and the overlap between tasks carried out by nurses and technicians. The possibility of overlap in other areas is evident, with increasing interest and concern on the part of professional bodies and organizations about the developing role of the advanced nurse practitioner. The concern and interest essentially spring from two different points of view: one focused on the changing scope of the nurse's professional practice (UKCC 1992); the other focused on the possibility of nurse practitioners taking on clinical duties normally assigned to junior medical staff in training (Higginson 1992; DoH 1993; Greenhalge and Company 1994).

The nurse practitioner role has been taken on by nurses in the community (Stilwell *et al.* 1987; Drury *et al.* 1988) and is being initiated in a wide range of hospital specialities, including cardiovascular surgery, urology, paediatrics, and accident and emergency care. In the area of neonatal nursing, an advanced practitioner course has been set up in one English health region (Hall *et al.* 1991).

The study

As part of a large-scale national study of neonatal nursing, commissioned and funded by the Department of Health, London (Redshaw *et al.* 1993a,b), the issue of the changing role of the neonatal nurse was addressed. In general, the study aimed to document many aspects of the working environment of neonatal units, focusing on a wide range of organizational and individual factors. The first stage involved the collection of general information from a large number of neonatal units, the second concerned the work, perceptions and experiences of a large number of individual nurses, and the third stage involved participation of parents whose babies had been in neonatal care.

Specifically in relation to the 'extended' and 'expanding' role of the neonatal nurse, the aim was to assess the ways in which nurses in neonatal care had already begun to change their role, the effects of grade and qualification in specialty (QIS) on these aspects of practice, and nurses' attitudes to these professional developments.

Methods

The results presented below arise from the data collection that took place during the second stage of the study. Four neonatal units in each of six health regions in England were visited (a regional centre, a subregional centre and two district units), resulting in a total of 24 study sites. The definitions of the types of unit are as found in the Report of the Royal College of Physicians (1988). The units were selected to provide a widely distributed, and yet representative, sample in terms of size, location and the population served.

All nursing staff involved in caring for babies or directly responsible for neonatal unit management were invited to participate. Following ethical committee permission, staff lists were obtained from senior nurses or managers. Each unit was visited, and individually addressed letters and questionnaires were left for each nurse to complete and return directly. Nonresponders were contacted again 4 weeks later, but not subsequently.

Throughout the study confidentiality was of the utmost importance. Rigorous professional guidelines were followed: numbered questionnaires were used, data were made anonymous and entered on the project computer system, and data in any form are only accessible to the research team. At each hospital visit, during which nurses on the different shifts were seen, these points were stressed to the nurses being asked to participate.

Sample

A total of 929 nurses were recruited to the study, of whom 718 (78%) returned complete questionnaires. The questionnaire itself covered a wide range of topics, including education, training and experience and health. It also contained a large section about the current working situation. Senior nurses were interviewed at the time of the visit and data were obtained concerning unit policy on the role of nursing staff in neonatal care. In order to address the question of how far the 'extended' or 'expanded' role was in operation in this specialty, nurses were questioned using a list of 30 tasks. These included methods of blood sampling, administration of drugs, and a wide range of technical and invasive procedures. Nurses were asked whether they had undertaken the task in the past and whether they were doing so regularly now. If they had not yet carried out the task, they were asked whether they wished to do so. This area of the task inventory was in addition to the data collection on more traditional aspects of neonatal care nursing.

The data presented are those obtained from 599 qualified nurses in the D–I grades, unless otherwise indicated. In examining the effects of grade, unit type and qualification in specialty on the performance of specific tasks, the appropriate χ^2 test was used.

Results

Policy on the expanded role of the nurse

Interviews with unit nursing managers indicated that for a quarter of units (six out of 24) there was a policy regarding the expanded role of the nurse. The units with such a policy comprised two regional centres, one subregional centre and three district units.

When asked about specific activities, heelprick blood sampling was reported for all units, administration of intravenous (IV) antibiotics for 88% (21 units) and removal of intravenous cannulae for 83% (20 units). Intravenous administration of other drugs at 67% (16 units), intubation at 42% (10 units), use of a blood gas analyser at 63% (15 units) and use of a bilirubinometer at 42% (10 units) were less common. No unit managers reported nursing staff undertaking insertion of intra-arterial (IA) cannulae, umbilical arterial catheters (UAC) or chest drains.

Tasks commonly undertaken by individual nurses

The individual data collected show that those tasks routinely carried out by nurses working in neonatal care and graded D–I include: taking heelprick blood samples (90%), removing IV cannulae (89%), and giving IV antibiotics (67%). Higher proportions of nurses had actually carried out these tasks at some time, but were not doing so regularly: 98% heelprick sampling, 98% removing IV cannulae, and 77% giving IV antibiotics.

The distribution of tasks carried out by nurses grade D–I is presented in Fig. 11.1, showing a significant effect for the giving of IV antibiotics ($P < 0.001$), but little difference on the other tasks shown. When these data are displayed according to unit type (Fig. 11.2), few differences are evident.

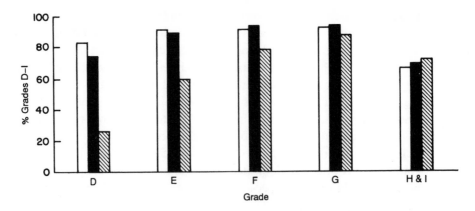

Fig. 11.1   Common tasks carried out regularly by neonatal nurses at different grades. ☐ heelprick, ■ remove intravenous cannula, ▧ give intravenous antibiotics. Source: Neonatal Nurses Project (DoH 1993).

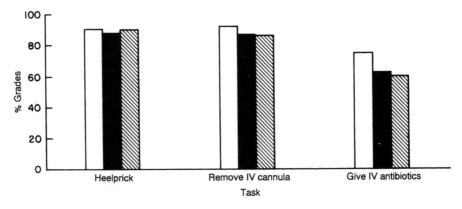

Fig. 11.2   Common tasks carried out regularly by neonatal nurses in different types of unit. ☐ regional, ■ subregional, ▧ district. Source: Neonatal Nurses Project (DoH 1993).

Less common activities

Other less common tasks and areas of care that some nurses working in neonatal units appeared to be taking on were examined. Intravenous administration of drugs other than antibiotics was regularly undertaken by 50% of nurses, removal of endotracheal (ET) tubes (as an emergency or elective procedure) by 44%, setting up of arterial blood-pressure monitoring by 41%, and removal of peripheral IA cannulae by 38%. As with the more common tasks, greater numbers of nurses had carried these out previously, though were not doing them on a regular basis now. At some time 65% of nurses had given drugs other than antibiotics intravenously, 80% had removed ET tubes, 66% had set up arterial BP monitoring, and 66% had removed peripheral IA cannulae.

Differences across the grades in carrying out these tasks are shown in Fig. 11.3. There is a clear effect of seniority, with significantly more G grades regularly undertaking these tasks than nurses at any of the other levels ($P < 0.01$–0.001).

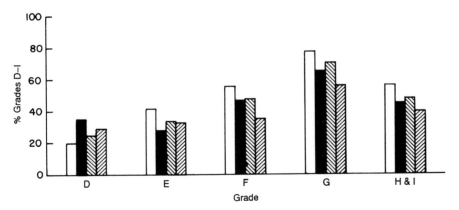

Fig. 11.3   Less common tasks carried out regularly by neonatal nurses. □ other drugs (intravenously), ■ set up blood-pressure monitoring, ▨ remove endotracheal tube, ▨ remove intra-arterial cannula. Source: Neonatal Nurses Project (DoH 1993).

Differences according to unit type are shown in Fig. 11.4. The proportion of nurses carrying out these tasks was greatest in the regional centres, followed by the subregional and then the district units ($P < 0.001$), reflecting both the levels of care available and the type of babies admitted.

Other still less common tasks that were regularly carried out by 20% or less of D–I grades were: removal of an umbilical arterial catheter (20%), using a blood gas analyser (13%), using a bilirubinometer (12%), and taking

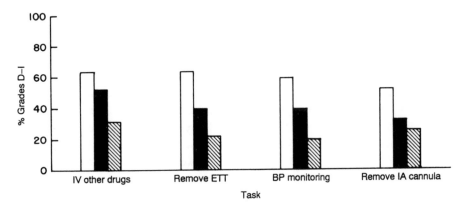

Fig. 11.4   Less common tasks carried out regularly by neonatal nurses in different types of unit. □ regional, ■ subregional, ▨ district. Source: Neonatal Nurses Project (DoH 1993).

a blood sample from an indwelling arterial catheter (9%). A frequency distribution by grade is shown in Fig. 11.5. Similar significant effects of grade to those reported for more common tasks were found ($P < 0.01$) for all except use of a bilirubinometer. Some less obvious effects of unit type were found; for example, the use of a bilirubinometer was actually higher for nurses working in subregional and district units (21% and 19% compared with 2% in regional centres).

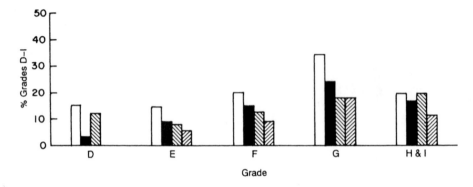

Fig. 11.5   Other less common tasks carried out regularly by neonatal nurses. □ remove UAC, ■ blood gas analyser, ◩ use bilirubinometer, ▨ sample intra-arterial catheter. Source: Neonatal Nurses Project (DoH 1993).

The tasks that were most infrequently reported as a routine part of the neonatal nurse's work are shown in Table 11.1. It appears that a small proportion of nurses in neonatal care are carrying out these and other tasks that have more usually been carried out by medical staff. It is also clear that some nurses have previously performed tasks that they are not currently undertaking.

Nurses with a specialist qualification

In general, more nurses with a specialist qualification were carrying out the tasks examined than those without a post-registration neonatal nursing qualification. However, for the two most common activities (heelprick samplings and removing IV cannulae), being QIS made little difference. Of all the staff carrying out heelpricks, 48% were QIS and the comparable figure for nurses removing IV cannulae was 51%. For all the other tasks examined, including the giving of antibiotics intravenously, there was a significant relationship with having a post-registration neonatal qualification ($P < 0.001$ for all but use of the blood gas analyser and the bilirubinometer, for which the values were $P < 0.01$ and $P < 0.02$ respectively). The proportion of QIS nurses undertaking the less common tasks was quite high and

Table 11.1 Tasks carried out infrequently by neonatal nurses, grades D–I ($n = 599$) (in percentages).

Tasks	Nurses carrying out task regularly	Nurses having carried out task previously
Venepuncture	1.17	12.19
Arterial stab	0.33	1.50
Insertion of intravenous cannula	1.67	11.02
Insertion of intra-arterial cannula	0.33	0.67
Insertion of umbilical arterial catheters	0.17	0.50
Insertion of central venous pressure catheter	0.17	0.17
Intubation	1.67	21.54
Insertion of chest drain	0.50	1.00
Removal of chest drain	4.84	24.87
Lumbar puncture	0.17	0.17
Calculation of total parenteral nutrition requirements	0.50	3.84

varied relatively little between the tasks, ranging from 61% of nurses using a bilirubinometer to 75% of those taking a blood sample from an indwelling arterial catheter.

Junior (A–C) grade staff

Data were also collected from the more junior (A–C) grade staff on the same range of tasks. Of the 119 staff in the study at these grades, all were nursery nurses or nursing auxiliaries except nine who were enrolled nurses. Heelprick blood sampling had been carried out by more than 80% of the staff at these grades; 52% had removed an IV cannula and 15% had used a bilirubinometer. More rarely, some staff at these grades had undertaken administration of IV antibiotics, removal of an ET tube, removal of an IA cannula, and use of a blood gas analyser. Using nurses at these grades for these tasks was not found to be restricted to any particular type of unit.

Attitudes to the changing role

Many D–I grade nurses expressed interest in expanding their role in neonatal care. The majority of nurses who had not carried out the most common tasks wished to do so as part of their current practice: heelprick blood sampling (eight out of the 10), removal of an IV cannula (seven out of the 11) and giving IV antibiotics (104 out of 138). With the less common tasks, 51% of the nurses who had not already done so would like to be able to give drugs, other than antibiotics, intravenously; 63% would like to site IV cannulae, 71% to intubate, 40% to remove ET tube, 63% to use a bilirubinometer and 74% to use a blood gas analyser.

Much smaller numbers of nurses would like to perform a lumbar puncture (8%), insert a chest drain (9%) or insert an umbilical arterial catheter (16%).

Discussion

It seems that some of the tasks examined have already been incorporated into the day-to-day work of nurses in neonatal care. The data collected on policy and practice appear to agree in relation to the most common tasks examined. Thus heelprick blood sampling, removal of an IV cannula and giving IV antibiotics are part of the skill base commonly expected of qualified and trained nurses working in this specialty.

Areas of skill involving more invasive procedures, the use of advanced technical equipment, or in which decision-making is an integral part, clearly have yet to be accepted as part of the role on a broad scale. In a small number of units, though the stated policy was for nurses not to take on such tasks, they were in fact doing so as a regular part of their work. This, and the use of unqualified and untrained staff to carry out technical nursing tasks, raises questions about the legal implications of these aspects of practice and the extent of liability assumed by the employing authority. To argue that such untrained staff are 'supervised' while carrying out these tasks is unacceptable, in view of the high levels of expertise demanded in post-registration course training and the realities of supervision. The use of unqualified staff as nurses working in this way in an acute specialty like neonatal care cannot be regarded as good practice.

The lower levels of practice found for H and I grades, on both the common and less common tasks examined, probably reflect a reduced level of clinical involvement and more commitment in the spheres of management or teaching for some individuals.

Changes in policy and practice

Changes in policy, differences in experience and the practice of different units may account for the large frequency differences found between the relatively low proportion of nurses regularly carrying out certain tasks (for instance venepuncture or removal of a chest drain), and the higher proportion who have carried out these tasks at some time previously. For the nurse who has learnt new skills, moving to another unit may mean no longer being able to practice them. Local certification may be useful in the short term to both employer and employee, but variations in policy and training both within and between hospitals render them unsatisfactory.

Unit type differences in practice of the kind described are probably a function of medical staffing and cover as well as of nursing policy developments. Thus, where there are fewer numbers of junior doctors or where medical cover is generally poor, nurses may have taken on duties that in other circumstances would not have been considered within their area of expertise. Concerns about the quality of care given to babies have led nurses to consider taking on additional tasks, despite staffing inadequacies and the absence of a planned career structure (Redshaw *et al.* 1993c). Educational training programmes, orientation, assessment of competence, and updating of skills are all required elements in preparation for major professional developments of this kind.

Role developments

The findings, supported by observations made during study visits, are based on a task-oriented approach to nursing developments in neonatal care. This approach facilitated accurate data collection and enabled a detailed profile of current practice to be constructed. However, from many perspectives the changing role of the neonatal nurse is as much a function of changing perceptions of the nursing and medical interface as of the specific activities employed in the role. To many neonatal nurses, the changing role should include areas such as training, education, research, and family-centred care.

The evidence from the present study of nurses working in neonatal units is that there are some areas of activity which they see as part of their job and others they would like to take on, given appropriate training and recognition. However, there are some technically difficult and invasive tasks which relatively few nurses wish to encompass in their role.

Findings from the study are of direct relevance to many of the currently proposed developments and new models of care in the organization and provision of neonatal services. The information collected and presented could provide a context and point for comparison against which to view these and other future developments.

Acknowledgements

The study was commissioned and funded by the Department of Health, London, but the opinions expressed are those of the researchers alone. Thanks are due to Jenny Ingram, Tina Owen, and Mike Taysum for data input and computing, and to the project advisory group for support and advice. Most of all, we would like to acknowledge the large number of nurses working in neonatal care who willingly participated in the study.

References

Audit Commission (1993) *Children First*. HMSO, London.

Beresford, D. (1991) Neonatal nurse practitioners in Canada and Sweden. Unpublished report to Nottingham Neonatal Services, Queens Medical Centre, Nottingham, October.

Boxall, J. (1987) The Development of Neonatal Nurse Practitioners. Paper presented at the Neonatal Nurses Association Annual Conference, Nottingham.

Chiswick, M. & Roberton, N.(1987) Doctors and nurses in neonatal care: towards integration. *Archives of Disease in Childhood*, **62**, 653–5.

Department of Health (1989) *Survey of Nurses in High Technology Care*. Department of Health, London.

Department of Health, Working Group on Specialist Medical Training (1993) *Hospital Doctors: Training for the Future*. Health Publications Unit, Oldham, Lancashire.

Drury, M., Greenfield, S., Stilwell, B. & Hull, F. (1988) A nurse practitioner in general practice: patient perceptions and expectations. *Journal of The Royal College of General Practitioners*, **38**(316), 503–5.

Greenhalge and Company (1994) *The Interface Between Junior Doctors and Nurses*. A research study for the Department of Health. Greenhalge & Company Limited, Macclesfield, Cheshire.

Hale, P., Boxall, J. & Hunt, M. (1987) The role of the neonatal nurse practitioner: a viewpoint. *Archives of Disease in Childhood*, **62**, 760–61.

Hall, M., Smith, S. & Jackson, J. (1991) Neonatal Nurse Practitioners: The Way Forward. Origins and Development of the Wessex Initiative. The Challenge of Caring '91 Conference, Vickers, London.

Hall, M., Smith, S., Jackson, J., Perks, E. & Walton, P. (1992) Neonatal nurse practitioners: a view from Perfidious Albion? *Archives of Disease in Childhood*, **67**, 458–62.

Harvey, D., Cooke, R.W.I. & Levitt, G. (eds) (1989) *The Baby Under 1000 g*. Wright, London.

Herbert, F. & Little, C. (1983) Nurse Practitioner Program, University of Alberta. *Canadian Medical Association Journal*, **128**(11), 1311–12.

Higginson, I. (1992) *Description and Preliminary Evaluation of Department of Health Initiatives To Reduce Junior Doctors' Hours*. Report for the NHS Management Executive, Department of Health, London.

Karp, T. (1993) *Neonatal Nursing: Pathway To Excellence or A Dead End Profession?* Neonatal Nurses Association Conference, Nottingham.

Redshaw, M.E., Harris, A. & Ingram, J.C. (1993a). The neonatal unit as a working environment: a survey of neonatal unit nursing. Unpublished report to the Department of Health, London.

Redshaw, M.E., Harris, A. & Ingram, J.C. (1993b) *The Neonatal Unit as a Working Environment: A Survey of Neonatal Unit Nursing* (Executive Summary). Department of Health, London.

Redshaw, M.E., Harris, A. & Ingram, J.C. (1993c) Nursing and medical staffing in neonatal units. *Journal of Nursing Management*, **1**(5), 221–8.

Roberton, N.R.C. (1993) *A Manual of Neonatal Intensive Care*, 3rd edn. Edward Arnold, Sevenoaks, Kent.

Royal College of Physicians (1988) *Medical Care of the Newborn in England and Wales*. RCP, London.

Stilwell, B., Greenfield, S., Drury, M. & Hull, F. (1987) A nurse practitioner in general practice. *Journal of The Royal College of General Practitioners*, **37**(297), 154–7.

Stock, J. & Ball, J. (1992) *A Study of Nurses and Technicians in High Technology Areas*. Institute of Manpower Studies, Brighton.

United Kingdom Central Council on Nursing, Midwifery and Health Visiting (1992) *The Scope of Professional Practice*. UKCC Position Statement. UKCC, London.

Youngman, M., Mockett, S. & Baxter, C. (1988) *The Roles of Nurses and Technicians in High Technology Clinical Areas: A Preliminary Report*. Department of Health and Social Security, London.

Chapter 12
Parents, nurses and paediatric nursing: a critical review

PHILIP DARBYSHIRE, *RNMH, RSCN, DipN, RNT, MN, PhD*

Senior Lecturer in Health and Nursing Studies, Department of Health and Nursing Studies, Glasgow Caledonian University, Glasgow, Scotland

The desirability of encouraging parents to live-in with their hospitalized child is widely accepted (DoH 1991). This review traces the historical development of parental involvement in paediatrics. The literature reviewed shows that parental participation and living-in has been viewed largely as philosophically and professionally unproblematic. These 'cardinal principles' of paediatric nursing have been advocated and operationalized with little or no attempt made to understand what living-in is like for either parents or for the nurses who work with them. It is proposed that research approaches in this area are required which are more hermeneutic and dialogic.

Introduction

Hospitalization has long been recognized as a potentially stressful experience for both children and their parents. Since the publication of the Platt Report on the welfare of children in hospital (Ministry of Health and Central Health Services Council 1959), there have been various attempts to humanize paediatric hospitals by offering open visiting (Fagin & Nusbaum 1978), living-in facilities for parents (Hardgrove 1980), and by encouraging parents to take a more active part in their hospitalized child's care (Cleary *et al.* 1986; Sainsbury *et al.* 1986).

However, there is evidence to suggest that while such changes may be desirable, their implementation has been more difficult than was first imagined (Hall 1978; Consumers' Association 1980; Hall 1987). Hospitals are complex environments, and the phrase 'encourage parents to live-in with their child' tends to understate the implications, for both parents and paediatric nurses, of this increased parental presence (Elfert & Anderson 1987; Hall 1987).

Throughout the literature on paediatric hospitalization there is a lack of detailed description of how parents and nurses perceive these changes. The questions 'How do parents experience living-in with their child in a paediatric ward?' and 'What is the nature of nurses' relationships with live-in parents?' remained unexplored until relatively recently (Knafl *et al.* 1988; Thorne & Robinson 1988 a,b; Darbyshire 1992).

This chapter focuses selectively upon those aspects of paediatric hospitalization which reflect parents' and nurses' experiences, particularly where this relates to parents who live-in with their child. It begins by outlining the changes in philosophies of paediatric care which have taken place this century. This provides a context within which to discuss the more germane aspects of parental living-in, parental involvement and participation in the child's care, and the nature of the nurse–parent relationship.

The historical context

Hospitals for sick children are relatively new institutions, emerging mainly in the mid-nineteenth century (Miles 1986, a,b). Prior to this there existed dispensaries which gave advice and medicine to parents who called. The first of these was opened by Dr George Armstrong in 1769. Dr Armstrong believed that children should not be separated from their parents and admitted to hospital, claiming prophetically that, 'the mothers and the nurses would be constantly at variance with each other' (Miles 1986a).

The early struggle against infectious diseases and often fatal illnesses helped to create a hospital system based upon asepsis and rigid following of routine. The legacy of this system was to affect the relationships between children, parents and hospital staff for over a century and its last vestiges may even be apparent today.

The ethos of child care within the paediatric hospitals was not shaped solely by physical and epidemiological factors. The child-rearing ideologies of the early twentieth century provided further justification for mechanistic and regimented care. Hardyment (1983) showed that the prevailing orthodoxy of the time regarding relationships with children was one of firm, cold detachment. Child care experts of the 1920s and 1930s such as Truby King and J.B. Watson advocated the strictest adherence to 'by-the-clock' behaviourist routines, which eschewed emotional interaction with the child as essentially 'mawkish' and 'sentimental' (Hardyment 1983).

With the decline in infectious diseases, and the introduction of antibiotics and technological innovations, these patterns of child care might have been expected to disappear. However, changes in thinking concerning the child's psychological and emotional development were to be the most effective catalysts for change.

The work of Bowlby and Robertson

Many view the watershed events regarding care of the hospitalized child as being the work of Bowlby (1953) and Robertson (1962, 1970). Bowlby's highly influential work on 'maternal deprivation' was seen as being particularly applicable to the situation of the hospitalized child. The Robertsons' films of children undergoing hospitalization and separation had a dramatic effect on professional and public opinion, as viewers were confronted with the sight of the emotional disintegration of children in places whose ostensible purpose was to help them. The impact of films such as *John: Nine Days in a Residential Nursery*, and *A Two Year Old Goes to Hospital*, was enhanced by the Robertsons' stark, almost telegrammatic commentary, which attracted criticism from professionals for being 'subjective' (Hawthorne 1974). However, such critics declined to suggest how the documentary of a child's pain and distress could be commented upon objectively.

During this period, some paediatric nurses began to advocate more humane and family-focused practices, such as allowing parents to visit their hospitalized child. Duncombe (1951) wrote of the 'arguments against daily visiting which I hear again and again both in personal conversation and at professional meetings'. In the present era, it is difficult to comprehend that the position which she was defending against such entrenched criticism was that of allowing parents to visit their child for 'one planned half-hour a day'. A *Nursing Times* (1953) editorial of the time was similarly critical of the restrictions which kept parents and their children apart. It noted that:

'In the Annual Report for the Ministry (of Health) for 1952, tables showed that 141 hospitals under regional hospital boards and three teaching hospitals prohibited the visiting of children except in emergency.'

At this time paediatric nurses in the USA were also describing how they were influenced by psychological theories of separation, and how they were trying to encourage contact between hospitalized children and their parents (Frank 1952; Morgan & Lloyd 1955; Hartrich 1956; Hohle 1957).

The Platt Report

The major impetus towards reuniting parents with their hospitalized child came with the publication of the Platt Report (Ministry of Health and Central Health Services Council 1959), and in subsequent Ministry of Health memoranda, which stressed the importance of open visiting. The central thrust of the Platt Report was that greater heed had to be taken of the hospitalized child's emotional and psychological welfare. This was to be achieved through the report's major recommendations. These were: that alternatives to in-patient treatment should be available; that children should be admitted to children's hospitals or wards; that children's nurses should be specifically trained; that parents should be able to visit at any 'reasonable' time of day or night; and that organized play and recreational activities should be provided in each ward.

Implementation of the Platt Report

The fate of the Platt Report is perhaps best understood in the light of Florence Nightingale's famous observation that 'reports are not necessarily self-executive'. Progress in implementing the recommendations of the Platt Report was slow and varied greatly across the country (Consumers' Association 1980; Rodgers 1980; Swanwick 1983). Government action was limited to the issuing of a succession of circulars which only 'advised'. Sixteen years after Platt, the Court Report (DHSS 1976) was able to note that:

> 'A great deal of evidence we received underlined the fact that it is in the sphere of social understanding of their needs that the children are least well cared for ... our visits made it clear that the personal needs of children in acute hospitals were not being met.'

In 1961 a group of parents formed NAWCH (National Association for the Welfare of Children in Hospital), now called Action for Sick Children. Since then NAWCH has monitored and reported on how the spirit and the recommendations of the Platt Report were being put into practice throughout the country. In relation to parental access to children, NAWCH reported that, in England, children were still being admitted to adult and paediatric ENT wards where visiting restrictions were greater than in general paediatric wards (Thornes 1983a). Thornes (1983b) also found wide variations in access, for example unrestricted access was allowed in only 21% of wards in the Northern Region, compared with 82% in the North East Thames Region. In a similar Scottish study, Wolfe (1985) found that unrestricted access for parents was claimed for 61% of wards, although in 9% parental visits on operating day were restricted. Sixteen of the wards could not or would not accommodate parents overnight.

Limitations of the Platt Report

Hall (1978) argued that the slow and piecemeal implementation of the Platt Report's recommendations was due to the fact that Platt had considered only psychological theory, that is, mother–child separation. The report had ignored, Hall believed, the wider sociological implications of hospitals as institutions, and the difficulty inherent in effecting change within such places. Hall (1978) also argued that having parents in the ward, as visitors or residents, created resistance from staff who did not accept that parents should be there. Nor did staff accept the evidence which suggested that parental presence was a good thing.

There seemed little doubt that the Platt Report's analyses of the problem and suggested solutions were rather narrow in vision and naive in expectation. Parents were encouraged to stay with their child during hospitalization, either as 'long-term' and regular visitors or as residents. What had not been seriously considered was how parents and nurses would experience this living-in, what would be expected of them and what effect such living-in would have upon their child care and nursing practices, respectively.

Parental involvement and participation

The literature on parental participation, from both the UK and North America, suggests that this is one of paediatric nursing's most amorphous and ill-described concepts. Parents and nurses seem to have different attitudes toward the concept, different ideas as to what the term actually means and different notions as to what parental participation involves within the setting of the daily life of a children's ward.

In an influential study Meadow (1969, 1974) described the lives of live-in parents under the graphic title of *The Captive Mother*. He suggested that such parents were akin to prisoners in that they were confined, not by bars but by expectations and a sense of anomie. The parents described their situation as being primarily one of boredom, where their role was merely to sit by the bedside while having little or no involvement in their child's care.

Several other studies at this time showed that mothers were keen to have a more active participatory role in the care of their child. Beck (1973) surveyed 38 parents to ascertain their attitudes towards a 'patient care unit', or what would now be called a 'care by parent unit' (Monaghan & Schkade 1985; Sainsbury *et al.* 1986), where parents have responsibility for providing their child's daily care with guidance and support available from nurses.

While the parents felt comfortable about carrying out aspects of care such as emotional support, accompanying the child for tests, and feeding and changing, they were unsure as to their own ability to carry out more technical or procedural care, such as the recording of vital signs or helping to administer medications. The reasons which they gave for this suggested a compromised self-confidence and sense of competence. They were unwilling to upset the hospital routine and 'get in the way' and were also wary of making a mistake.

Jackson *et al.* (1978) sought to determine parents' desire for participation at the time of their child's admission to hospital, with a view to sharing this information with the ward nursing staff. Of the 31 parents questioned, 'the overwhelming majority wanted to participate in their child's care, and for the most part they wanted to do so without the aid of a nurse'.

Preferred areas of care

An earlier study by Merrow & Johnson (1968) suggested discrepancies between mothers and paediatric nurses regarding 'what a mother would like her own role to be with her hospitalized child'. The researchers concluded that 'in most instances the mothers preferred to be responsible for more aspects of their child's care than the paediatric nurses realized'. This finding has been supported by other studies, for example Webb *et al.* (1985) and more recently, Brown & Ritchie (1990).

Several studies found that parents were generally keen to participate and be involved in their child's care. In a study of 76 parents of non-seriously ill children, McDonald (1969) found that over 90% of the parents were willing to carry out nurturing, encouraging and washing and feeding tasks. While mothers were willing to participate in various areas of care, Hawthorne (1974), for example, found that nurses were much more inclined to encourage parents to become involved in 'basic nursing tasks' (*sic*) such as washing, feeding and changing the child. Hawthorne (1974) also reported an 'overwhelming reluctance' on the part of nurses to allow parents to participate in any nursing care which 'might be described in any way as technical nursing'.

Hill (1978) interviewed 18 mothers, regarding their participation in four categories of care: stimulation entertainment, comfort measures, activities of daily living and therapeutic measures. It was found that 78% of the mothers, overall, wanted to participate in their child's care. Hill noted that over 90% of the mothers wanted to participate mainly in comfort and stimulation entertainment work, while only 61% were keen to become involved in more technical medical routines.

Information for parents regarding their role

Algren (1985) studied 20 parents to discover not only the areas of care in which they participated but how much information they had been given by nurses regarding their role during their child's stay. A total of 40% of the parents were unsure as to whether they had been asked about this by staff and 60% said that they had 'definitely not' been consulted. It was reported by 70% that nurses had not discussed the role that they might or should adopt while living-in on the ward and 30% felt that this had been vaguely alluded to. All of the parents in this study wished to participate in their child's care, again especially in areas such as changing, feeding and comforting, as opposed to more technical procedural tasks.

Actual areas of parental involvement

Stull & Deatrick (1986) used semi-structured interviews and encouraged parents to keep a diary in an attempt to discover 'more specific activities pertaining to parental involvement during a child's hospitalization'. It was found that the majority of parental activities were 'direct care activities', such as physical care and comforting. The researchers also identified as being important, areas of parental activity where parents were not directly involved in 'hands-on' care of their child. These were areas such as discussing the child with staff and spending time with other parents or alone.

The majority of studies regarding parent participation have focused on mothers. This is not surprising in view of the fact that it is usually mothers rather than fathers who stay in with their child during hospitalization, although fathers have been playing a larger part in child care in recent years (Knafl & Dixon 1984).

Parents viewed as performers of tasks

Most commonly the discourse within the professional literature on parental involvement and participation centres around parents as performers of tasks which they will undertake in order to feel useful. Parents have been expected to feel that they were being useful both to their child and to the hospital. Meadow (1969) exemplified this understanding when he proposed that:

'Nurses must be trained in how to share care with a resident mother and how to use her as an efficient and willing source of labour.'

Similarly, Hawthorne (1974) noted that in one ward in her study, a visiting hours information slip stated that:

'We would appreciate it if parents of younger children would visit at appropriate meal times in order to feed children when possible.'

Again, in a more recent study, Keane *et al.* (1986), rather than supporting the idea that all children and parents could benefit from being together during hospitalization, suggested a need to 'clarify the characteristics of mothers and children most likely to benefit from residential facilities', since these parents 'are users of resources'.

Research omissions

The literature, described above, on parental participation exemplifies a technological and instrumental understanding of the person (Benner 1985; Taylor 1985) which is ultimately objectifying, and which may have helped to ensure that other ways of understanding parents' and nurses' experiences have been overlooked.

Specifically, despite carrying out several manual and computerized literature searches as part of a larger project in this area (Darbyshire 1992), the present author was unable to discover studies which had sought to understand the lived experience of resident parents' participation from a more phenomenological perspective.

A further omission in much of the literature on parent participation is that consideration of the situation within which participation occurs seems neglected in favour of isolating context-free variables. For example, studies which acknowledge the influence of nurses on parents' participation have focused on nurses' attitudes in relation to their place of work, level of education and rank (Seidl & Pilliterri 1967; Seidl 1969; Goodell 1979; Gill 1987a, b). Such studies addressed neither nurses' lived experiences of participating in care with resident parents nor the nature of their ongoing practices as related to parental participation and involvement. Additionally, no attempt was made to explore the meanings that the summary phrase 'parent participation' has for nurses. In order to see how previous researchers and writers have examined this wider situation, it is necessary to now consider the nurse–parent relationship.

Nurses and live-in parents

While nurses welcomed many of the Platt Report's recommendations, such as the need for children's nurses to have specialist paediatric training, they were less enthusiastic about parents having virtually unrestricted access to the wards. In short, they appeared wary of the idea of parents participating on any other than nurses' terms. This was made clear (Anstice 1970) by one nurse who wrote that:

> '... it is a fact that, in the enthusiasm for open house for mothers, many of the problems this can present to medical and nursing staff tend to be overlooked. They are, after all, professionals in their field, and having amateurs around is, as one suggested, like having wives on board ship.'

The situation which developed in the post-Platt era could be described as one where the presence of parents was tolerated rather than actively encouraged and where parents were often resented and not positively valued. Early American studies pointed to parents being seen as 'a problem' for nurses (Moran 1963; Mahaffy 1964) and to the underlying and often open mutual resentment which existed between these two groups (Berman 1966).

A similar situation was reported in the UK by Brain & MacLay (1968) who carried out a controlled experiment in 'allowing' certain parents to live-in with their child during and after ENT surgery. At the end of the experiment the researchers noted of the nursing staff that: 'They were unanimous in their opinion that they preferred the children to be admitted on their own.'

The reasons given by the nurses were that they found it easier to carry out procedures when parents were not there, they were able to make more personal contact with the child in the parent's absence and that some mothers were 'difficult'. In contrast to these findings, Hawthorne (1974) noted that 84.5% of nurses interviewed for her study denied that mothers got in the way of nurses. However, she also found that only one of nine wards studied encouraged mothers to become resident.

This 'resistance at ward level to the admission of mothers or fathers' was also noted by Stacey *et al.* (1970) in the first of the 'Swansea studies' of children in hospital. In a later, related study, Hall (1977) noted that for nurses, 'Parents too, were a feature of the ward that was disliked'. In the final part of this group of studies, Stacey (1979) continued to find that 'parents tend still to be treated as outsiders and be tolerated rather than integrated', while Hall (1979) stated that 'One interesting feature to arise out of the questionnaires administered ... was the strong negative view of parents held by some nurses'.

Paediatric nurses had a rich vocabulary of disparagement for parents. The 'thick' mother seemed not to understand what is happening, the 'neurotic' mother worried about her child, the 'lazy' mother did not help enough and the 'troublemaker' did not seem to fit into the generally accepted mould of what a good live-in parent should be. Anstice (1970) was disarmingly honest in her description of 'some mothers':

> 'Some are a support to the child and a help to the nurse. Some, fussy and neurotic, manage to be neither. Some again are unbelievably stupid – or perhaps it is too easy to forget that they just do not know things that any nurse takes for granted.'

Features of research into parents in hospital

The sociological perspective

Much of the research on parents in hospital, and particularly the 'Swansea studies', is characterized by several noteworthy features. A pervasive sociological perspective led, the present author suggests, to the nurse–parent relationship being viewed through the lens of general sociological theory. Thus the parents' and nurses' experiences were filtered through theoretical screens of 'power and control', 'treatment and moral careers', 'ideologies' and Goffmanesque 'dramaturgy'. The results of such studies are no doubt of sociological interest. However, what was ignored or filtered out is equally worthy of study, particularly those meaningful and relational dimensions of the lived experience of parents and nurses.

Deficit mode thinking

A second major characteristic of the surveyed literature is its focus on what Benner (1984) calls 'deficit mode' thinking. This literature is almost uniformly critical of both nurses and hospitals. Nurses are cast in the role of agents of social control and parents seem no more than passive ciphers in an institutional conspiracy which seeks to control and oppress them (e.g. Beuf 1979). The language of social structures and of given theories has been placed like a template over the study situation, occluding a vision of the everyday meanings, practices and understandings which are more local and contextual.

To criticize this literature for its deficit mode thinking is not to suggest the existence of an idealized world where all professional practice is laudable and where all nurse–parent relationships are mutually successful and satisfying. It is rather to propose that certain theoretical frameworks and research approaches represent a search for detached theoretical knowledge which serves the interests of social engineering. While such perspectives seem all too ready to explain the social world, they are ill-equipped to recognize and describe aspects of both nurses' and parents' practices and experiences which may be more positive.

Pill (1970) for example, described an observational approach based upon a sociology of suspicion and a notion that a subject–object dichotomy is both inevitable and desirable. Within this approach, the researcher seemed merely a 'research tool', standing above rather than beside the participants, and reporting on 'the facts of the situation'. Significantly here, Pill (1970) expressed the need for not only a theoretical screen, but also a physical one:

> 'Ideally, of course a one-way screen or other device for concealment would have been desirable, but this is obviously impossible to arrange in the average ward.'

The attempt to understand nurse–patient relationships from this stance seems to have led to other oversights. For example, Pill (1970) also remarked that:

> 'In the nature of things, there are long stretches of time when the routine care has been done and the nurse is merely keeping an eye on things.'

Such a comment betrays a misunderstanding of the complexity of nursing. It is also testimony to the value of later work by Benner (1984, 1989) and MacLeod (1990) among others, who have uncovered the wealth of nursing expertise and caring practices which can be so easily glossed over by summary phrases such as 'routine care' and 'merely keeping an eye on things'.

The 'Swansea studies' and the sociological climate

The 'Swansea studies' can be better understood by considering their production within the sociological climate of the time. The late 1960s and 1970s were something of a 'golden age' for British sociology, highlighted by its expansion and popularity within higher education (Payne *et al.* 1981). Sociology became synonymous with the ability to uncover, expose and understand what was 'really happening' within society and its institutions. Sociological thinking was critical thinking, but with the emphasis firmly placed upon critical. It sought to produce a radical critique, and to unmask and explain the world in terms of whichever theoretical perspective was employed.

Significantly, for a growing and expanding profession, sociology was also careful to ensure that problems were cast in sociological terms in order that solutions could also be similarly defined. From this perspective, the analysis and proposed solutions of Stacey *et al.* (1970) and Hall & Stacey (1979) seem rather self-serving. They claimed that the problems of children and their parents in hospital required a sociological understanding, which led inevitably to their call for 'social scientists to be in interaction with doctors and nurses' (Stacey 1979) and for increased teaching of social sciences throughout all nursing and medical education. Strong's comments (1979) are particularly apposite in relation to these studies:

'Scepticism has considerable dramatic rewards. In writing in this fashion, sociologists both formulate themselves as members of some insightful and incorruptible elite and, at the same time, gain considerable pleasure by the exposure and thus potential overthrow of those whom they dislike.'

Qualitative research of Hayes & Knox

Of particular relevance to the question of parents in paediatrics was a further body of predominantly qualitative research studies, undertaken by Hayes & Knox and Robinson & Thorne in Canada, which focused on children with a long-term chronic illness. Knox & Hayes (1983) (also Hayes & Knox 1984) used a grounded theory approach to examine the experience of stress in 40 parents. It is unclear whether these parents were resident but Knox & Hayes did note that mothers spent more time in hospital than fathers and 'felt a need to be present'. These researchers hinted that parents experienced fundamental changes, mentioning those who spoke of their whole life changing, and parents who described how no one but another parent could really understand the nature of their experiences.

However, Hayes & Knox did not follow this ontological lead, preferring to develop an account of the parents' stress in terms of the discrepant perspectives which, they argued, existed between parents and health care staff. They also employed role theory to suggest that parents' stress experiences were related to changed perceptions of their role when their child was hospitalized.

These studies were important in focusing attention on the perspective of parents of hospitalized children and highlighted several salient aspects of parents' experiences. It is suggested here, however, that the adopted perspective of role theory and an essentially mechanistic view of stress based on the work of Selya (1976) and Scott *et al.* (1980), obscured much of the parents' personal meaning which these studies might have revealed.

Limitations of role theory

Role theory is premised on the dualistic assumption that our *being* is distinct from our social practices. From this basis it is perhaps inevitable that the meaning of being a parent in these studies came to be seen in terms of end-goals and the playing of a part with associated connotations of inauthenticity. The conclusions of these studies were not quite so trivializing, however, as Stacey's view (1970) that parents were unable to 'play the role of "mother-in-the-ward"'. More recent studies from a phenomenological perspective (Leonard 1991; Darbyshire 1992) strongly suggest that a parent's way of 'being-in-the-world' (Heidegger 1962) cannot be adequately captured in the objective language of roles, which suggests chosen ends rather than integrated sets of practices through which we interpret and understand ourselves and order our everyday activities (Dreyfus 1991).

A further limitation of Hayes & Knox's role perspective is that it concentrates upon only one group of 'actors', the parents, thus losing the sense of shared human being which marks out our everyday experience. The role of parent of a hospitalized child makes little sense in isolation from, say, the role of the paediatric nurse, because of the importance of shared understandings and common meanings.

The research of Robinson & Thorne

The research of Robinson & Thorne (1984) was also significant in relation to nurse–parent relationships in paediatrics. As part of the 'Health Care Relationships Project', qualitative interviews were carried out with families with an adult member who had cancer and families with a chronically ill child. Robinson & Thorne contended that relationships between health care professionals, patients and parents developed according to discernible, predictable stages. These were: 'naive trusting', 'disenchantment' and 'guarded alliance'. As their titles suggested, these stages were characterized by families' increasing disenchantment with the nature of their relationships with health care providers until the stage of 'guarded alliance' was reached. This stage was achieved when the parents and patients were more aware of professionals' limitations, and where their trust was reconstructed on the basis of a more active and informed stances (Robinson & Thorne 1984).

A major difficulty in assessing the plausibility of Robinson & Thorne's thesis is that the study and interpretative conclusions were presented with almost no supporting evidence in the form of interview data. While the researchers' thinking and ideas were well represented, the voices and accounts of the study participants remained largely unheard. The progression from 'naive trusting' to 'guarded alliance' seemed seductively reassuring. It suggested a forward moving, linear development which sits comfortably with western and traditional scientific understanding.

While the researchers cannot be held responsible for how other nurses may use this model of relationship development, there is a danger that nurses may seize on these labels of progression in order to designate rather than understand parents' lived experiences. For example, this author remembers being able to recite James Robertson's stages of a child's 'settling-in' to hospital, Kubler-Ross's stages of dying, the four stages of group formation and the stages of the nursing process. How great an insight or understanding these stages afforded is debatable. I suspect that what was achieved by this thinking in stages was in fact a distancing from the person and their lived experiences, for they were now at least partially hidden by a label.

A further difficulty in evaluating Robinson & Thorne's work is that there seemed to be some confusion as to the theoretical basis and research method used in the studies. In the original report of the 'Health Care Relationships Project', the researchers stated only that their theory was based on 'separate qualitative studies' (Robinson & Thorne 1984). In a later study, it was stated that:

> 'analysis relied upon the grounded theory method of qualitative research (Glaser & Strauss 1967) and resulted in the confirmation of a three-stage process of relationship evolutions.'

However, a different account of their theoretical approach was offered in another paper to which they referred. In this report, Thorne & Robinson (1988b) claimed that:

> 'The phenomenological paradigm of qualitative methodology directed both the process of constructing accounts with informant family members and analysis of the data that emerged.'

This seeming contradiction may indicate either a confusion as to the distinct nature of grounded theory and phenomenology, or an assumption that the two terms are somehow interchangeable.

Parents' accounts

A further body of important writing in relation to parents, nurses and paediatric hospitalization are parents' accounts of their experiences of visiting or living-in with their child. These accounts should not be viewed as being merely anecdotal, private or subjective, but as affording valuable insights into parents' lived experiences.

In the collection of solicited parents' letters compiled by Robertson (1962), parents described how much they valued being able to stay with their sick child and, alternatively, how distressing it was for parents who were forbidden from doing this. Significant features of these parents' letters were how grateful they were for what they believed was the 'privilege' of being allowed to live-in, and how they seemed prepared to tolerate almost any level of inconvenience and discomfort to this end.

Parents' feelings of disorientation, disordered time perception and 'unreality' during living-in were described by Turner (1984), Hilton (1982) and Beckett (1986). Many parents described intense feelings of guilt, anger, depression and physical exhaustion at various points of their living-in (Nolan 1981; Hilton 1982; Turner 1984; Beckett 1986; Smith 1987).

Relations with hospital staff

In their relations with hospital staff, parents described a gamut of emotions and involvement. Feelings of helplessness and uncertainty were described by Turner (1984) and Smith (1987), while an anonymous mother (1984) and Arango (1900) wrote of their feelings of being excluded from discussion and information about their child, and of having no one who genuinely understood their experience and needs. Webb (1977), Turner (1984) and Martin (1986) explained that they found everyday child care tasks strange and difficult to perform within the ward.

Some of these parents described their relationships with nurses, highlighting the value that they attached to nurses who were open, honest, informal, caring and willing to listen and talk (Khoo 1972; Turner 1984; Martin 1986; Beckett 1986; Smith 1987). However, parents also described encounters with staff whom they felt had been rude, abrupt, arrogant and unhelpful (Robertson 1962; Webb 1977; Hilton 1982; Turner 1984; Smith 1987).

Discussion

This review has focused on three bodies of literature concerning the historical development of current paediatric care philosophy: parental participation and involvement in their child's care, nurse–parent relationships, and parents' own accounts of their experiences.

Limitations of the reviewed literature

The historical development of paediatrics saw parents' expertise and knowledge of their child usurped by professionals. This related not only to the child's physical care, but also to what has become known as their emotional and psychological care. Ostensibly, the Platt Report was an attempt to counter this movement by advocating a greater sensitivity towards parent–child separation and greater parental involvement.

However, the slow and patchy implementation of the Platt Report's recommendations, especially in relation to parental living-in and involvement, indicated the considerable oversights which flawed the report. While the lack of a wider sociological perspective may have contributed to lack of progress in 'humanizing' paediatric care, such a perspective alone offers only a limited understanding of the lived experiences and meanings of resident parents and paediatric nurses.

The literature of parental involvement was notable for its basis in an instrumental and technological understanding of parents as being essentially of functional value. From this perspective, parents too readily became problems to be managed or resources to be more effectively used by ward staff. This literature also seemed content to leave the fundamental meaning of parent participation unexplored and unproblematic while opting to measure and to propose socially engineered solutions.

Studies which sought to explain the nurse–parent relationship tended to cloak the participants' personal and shared meanings in sociological concepts. The legitimacy of these labels was difficult to appraise due to the researchers' common practice of assigning them while offering the reader minimal supporting data, in the form of participants' accounts.

Parents' own accounts offered interesting insights, but most of those published were brief and tended to concentrate on the more dramatic emotions and events which parents experienced. These accounts often overlooked the meanings related to the more everyday nature of the parents' lived experiences and the practices which sustained this.

Importance of the lived experiences of parents and nurses

This review has shown that the lived experiences of parents and nurses have been largely overlooked in previous research. This has resulted in significant gaps in our understanding of how parents experience staying with their child in hospital and how parents' relationships with paediatric nurses develop. If paediatric nursing is to continue to advocate and develop a philosophy of care based upon mutuality and partnership with parents, then nurses need a deeper understanding of the nature of parents' experiences and how these relate to their own nursing practices.

An alternative to an instrumental understanding of parents and nurses is to consider the person as constituted by a web of relationship with others (Bellah *et al.* 1985; Taylor 1985; Dreyfus 1991). In this way the relational and contextual aspects of lived experiences and relationships may be uncovered and the voices of the research participants may be heard rather than assumed or ignored.

Acknowledgement

This work forms part of a larger doctoral study completed while the author was a Scottish Home and Health Department Nursing Research Training Fellow (Darbyshire 1994).

References

Algren, C.L. (1985) Role perception of mothers who have hospitalised children. *Children's Health Care*, **14**(1), 6–9.

Anonymous (1984) One mother's view. *The Practitioner*, **228**(1396), 960.

Anstice, E. (1970) 'Nurse, where's my mummy?' *Nursing Times*, **66**(48), 1513–18.

Arango, P. (1990) A parent's perspective: Making family centred care a reality. *Children's Health Care*, **19**(1), 57–62.

Beck, M. (1973) Attitudes of parents of pediatric heart patients towards patient care units. *Nursing Research*, **22**(4), 334–8.

Beckett, J. (1986) The parent's view. *American Association for Respiratory Care Times*, **11**(6), 66, 68.

Bellah, R.N., Masden, R., Sullivan, W.M., Swidler, A. & Tipton, S. (1985) *Habits of the Heart: Individualism and Commitment in American Life*. University of California Press, Berkeley.

Benner, P. (1984) *From Novice to Expert: Excellence and Power in Clinical Nursing*. Addison-Wesley, Menlo Park, California.

Benner, P. (1985) Preserving caring in an era of cost-containment, marketing and high technology. *Yale Nurse*, August, 12–20.

Benner, P. (1989) *The quest for control and the possibilities of care*. Paper presented at the Applied Heidegger Conference, Berkeley, California.

Berman, D.C. (1966) Pediatric nurses as mothers see them. *American Journal of Nursing*, **66**(11), 2429–31.

Beuf, A.H. (1979 *Biting off the Bracelet: A Study of Children in Hospital*. University of Pennsylvania Press, Pennsylvania.

Bowlby, J. (1953) *Child Care and the Growth of Love*. Penguin, Harmondsworth.

Brain, D.J. & MacLay, I. (1968) Controlled study of mothers and children in hospital. *British Medical Journal*, **1**, 278–80.

Brown, J. & Ritchie, J.A. (1990) Nurses' perceptions of parent and nurse roles in caring for hospitalised children. *Children's Health Care*, **19**(1), 28–36.

Cleary, J., Gray, O.P., Hall, D.J., Rowlandson, P.. & Sainsbury, C.P.Q. (1986) Parental involvement in the lives of children in hospital. *Archives of Disease in Childhood*, **61**(8), 779–87.

Consumers' Association (1980) *Children in Hospital: A Which? Campaign Report*. Consumers' Association, London.

Darbyshire, P. (1992) Parenting in public: a study of the experiences of parents who live-in with their hospitalised child, and of their relationships with paediatric nurses. Unpublished PhD thesis. University of Edinburgh, Edinburgh.

Darbyshire, P. (1994) *Living with a Sick Child in Hospital: Parent and Nurse Perspectives.* Chapman and Hall, London.

Department of Health (1991) *Welfare of Children and Young People in Hospital.* Her Majesty's Stationery Office, London.

Department of Health and Social Security (1976) *Fit For the Future* (The Court Report). HMSO, London.

Dreyfus, H.L. (1991) *Being in the World: A Commentary on Heidegger's 'Being and Time, Division 1'.* MIT Press, Cambridge, Massachusetts.

Duncombe, M.A. (1951) Daily visiting in children's wards. *Nursing Times,* **47,** 587–8.

Elfert, H. & Anderson, J.M. (1987) More than just luck: parents' views on getting good nursing care. *Canadian Nurse,* **83**(4), 14–17.

Fagin, C.M. & Nusbaum, J.G. (1978) Parental visiting privileges in pediatric units: a survey. *Journal of Nursing Administration,* **8,** 24–7.

Frank, R. (1952) Parents and the pediatric nurse. *American Journal of Nursing,* **52**(1), 76–7.

Gill, K.M. (1987a) Parent participation with a family health focus: nurses' attitudes. *Pediatric Nursing,* **13**(2), 94–6.

Gill, K.M. (1987b) Nurses' attitudes toward parent participation: personal and professional characteristics. *Children's Health Care,* **15**(3), 149–51.

Glaser, B.G. & Strauss, A.L. (1967) *The Discovery of Grounded Theory,* Aldine, Chicago.

Goodell, S.A. (1979) Perceptions of nurses toward parent participation on pediatric oncology units. *Cancer Nursing,* **2,** 38–46.

Hall, D.J. (1977) *Social Relations and Innovation: Changing the State of Play in Hospitals.* Routledge and Kegan Paul, London.

Hall, D.J. (1978) Bedside blues: the impact of social research on the hospital treatment of sick children. *Journal of Advanced Nursing,* **3**(1), 25–37.

Hall, D.J.(1979) On calling for order: aspects of the organisation of patient care. In *Beyond Separation: Further Studies of Children in Hospital* (eds D.J. Hall & M. Stacey). Routledge and Kegan Paul, London.

Hall, D.J. (1987) Social and psychological care before and during hospitalisation. *Social Science and Medicine,* **25**(6), 721–32.

Hall, D.J. & Stacey, M. (eds) (1979) *Beyond Separation: Further Studies of Children in Hospital.* Routledge & Kegan Paul, London.

Hardgrove, C. (1980) Helping parents on the paediatric ward: a report on a survey of hospitals with 'living-in' programs. *Pediatrician,* **9,** 220–23.

Hardyment, C. (1983) *Dream Babies: Child Care from Locke to Spock.* Jonathan Cape, London.

Hartrich, P. (1956) Parents and nurses work together. *Nursing Outlook,* **4**(3), 146–8.

Hawthorne, P.J. (1974) *Nurses – I want My Mummy!* Royal College of Nursing, London.

Hayes, V.E. & Knox, J.E. (1984) The experience of stress in parents of children hospitalised with long-term disabilities. *Journal of Advanced Nursing,* **9**(4), 333–41.

Heidegger, M. (1962) *Being and Time* (trans. J. Macquarrie & E. Robinson). Blackwell Publishers, Oxford.

Hill, C. (1978) The mother on the pediatric ward: insider or outlawed? *Pediatric Nursing,* **4**(5), 26–9.

Hilton, T. (1982) A shared experience. *World Medicine,* **18**(2), 26.

Hohle, B. (1957) We admit the parents too. *American Journal of Nursing,* **57**(7), 865–7.

Jackson, P., Bradham, R. & Burwell, H. (1978) Child care in the hospital – a parent staff partnership. *American Journal of Maternal Child Nursing,* **3,** 104–7.

Jacobs, R. (1979) The meaning of hospital: the denial of emotions. In *Beyond Separation: Further Studies of Children in Hospital* (eds D.J. Hall & M. Stacey). Routledge and Kegan Paul, London.

Keane, S., Garralda, M.E. & Keen, J.H. (1986) Resident parents during paediatric admissions. *International Journal of Nursing Studies,* **23**(3), 247–53.

Khoo, H. (1972) Rapport between parents and nurses in a children's ward. *Nursing Journal of Singapore,* **12**(1), 21–3.

Knafl, K.A. & Dixon, D.M. (1984) The participation of fathers in their child's hospitalisation.

Issues in Comprehensive Pediatric Nursing, **7**(4–5), 269–81.

Knafl, K.A., Cavallari, K.A. & Dixon, D.M. (1988) *Pediatric Hospitalisation: Family and Nurse Perspectives*. Scott, Foresman, Glenview, Illinois.

Knox, J.E. & Hayes, V.E. (1983) Hospitalisation of a chronically ill child: a stressful time for parents. *Issues in Comprehensive Pediatric Nursing*, **6**, 217–26.

Leonard, V.W. (1991) *The transition to parenthood of first time mothers with career commitments: an interpretive study*. Paper presented at the Qualitative Health Research Conference, Edmonton, Canada, February.

McDonald, E.M. (1969) Parents' preparation in care of the hospitalised child. *Canadian Nurse*, **65**, 37–9.

MacLeod, M.L.P. (1990) Experience in everyday nursing practice: a study of 'experienced' ward sisters. Unpublished PhD thesis. University of Edinburgh, Edinburgh.

Mahaffy, P.R. (1964) Nurse–parent relationships in living-in situations. *Nursing Forum*, **3**, 52–68.

Martin, M. (1986) Confidence not courage. *Intensive Care Nursing*, **2**(1), 20–22.

Meadow, S.R. (1969) The captive mother. *Archives of Diseases in Childhood*, **44**(3), 362–7.

Meadow, R. (1974) Children, mothers and hospital. *New Society*, **27**(592), 318–20.

Merrow, D.L. & Johnson, B.S. (1968) Perception of the mother's role with her hospitalised child. *Nursing Research*, **17**(2), 155–6.

Miles, I. (1986a) The emergence of sick children's nursing: part one, sick children's nursing before the turn of the century. *Nurse Education Today*, **6**(2), 82–7.

Miles, I. (1986b) The emergence of sick children's nursing: part two, efforts and achievements in the 20th century. *Nurse Education Today*, **6**(3), 133–8.

Ministry of Health and Central Health Services Council (1959) *The Welfare of Children in Hospital* (Platt Report). Her Majesty's Stationery Office, London.

Monaghan, G.H. & Schkade, J.K. (1985) Comparing care by parent and traditional nursing units. *Pediatric Nursing*, **11**(6), 463–8.

Moran, P.(1963) Parents in pediatrics. *Nursing Forum*, **2**(3), 24–37.

Morgan, M.L. & Lloyd, B.J. (1955) Parents invited. *Nursing Outlook*, **3**(5), 256–7.

Nolan, H. (1981) Hospitalisation of infants and pre-schoolers: observations and reflections by a live-in mother. *The Lamp*, **38**(8), 29–35.

Nursing Times (1953) Editorial: The child as a person in the hospital. *Nursing times*, **49**, 1153–4.

Payne, G., Dingwall, R., Payne, J. & Carter, M. (1981) *Sociology and Social Research*. Routledge and Kegan Paul, London.

Pill, R. (1970) The sociological aspects of the case-study sample. In *Hospitals, Children and Their Families* (ed M. Stacey). Routledge and Kegan Paul, London.

Robertson, J. (1962) *Hospitals and Children: A Review of Letters From Parents to 'The Observer' and the BBC*. Victor Gollancz, London.

Robertson, J. (1970) *Young Children in Hospital*, 2nd edn. Tavistock, London.

Robinson, C.A. & Thorne, S. (1984) Strengthening family 'interference'. *Journal of Advanced Nursing*, **9**(6), 597–602.

Rodgers, R. (1980) *From Crowther to Warnock: How 14 Reports Tried to Change Children's Lives*. Heinemann Educational Books, London.

Sainsbury, C.P.Q., Gray, O.P., Cleary, J., Davies, M.M. & Rowlandson, P.H. (1986) Care by parents of their children in hospital. *Archives of Disease in Childhood*, **61**(6), 612–15.

Scott, D.W., Oberst, M.T. & Dropkin, M.J. (1980) A stress-coping model. *Advances in Nursing Science*, **3**, 9–23.

Seidl, F.W. (1969) Pediatric nursing personnel and parent participation: a study in attitudes. *Nursing Research*, **18**(1), 40–44.

Seidl, F. & Pilliterri, A. (1967) Development of an attitude scale on parent participation. *Nursing Research*, **16**, 71–3.

Selye, H. (1976) *Stress in Health and Disease*. Butterworths, London.

Smith, S.M. (1987) Primary Nursing in the NICU: a parent's perspective. *Neonatal Network*, **5**(4), 25–7.

Stacey, M. (1979) The practical implications of our conclusions. In *Beyond Separation: Further*

Studies of Children in Hospital (eds D.J. Hall & M. Stacey). Routledge and Kegan Paul, London.

Stacey, M., Dearden, R. Pill, R. & Robinson, D. (1970) *Hospitals, Children and Their Families: The Report of a Pilot Study*. Routledge and Kegan Paul, London.

Strong, P.M. (1979) Sociological imperialism and the profession of medicine. *Social Science and Medicine*, **13A**, 199–215.

Stull, M.K. & Deatrick, J.A. (1986) Measuring parental participation: Part I. *Issues in Comprehensive Pediatric Nursing*, **9**(3), 157–65.

Swanwick, M. (1983) Platt in perspective. *Nursing Times*, Occasional Paper, **79**(2), 5–8.

Taylor, C. (1985) *Human Agency and Language: Philosophical Paper 1*. Cambridge University Press, Cambridge.

Thorne, S.E. & Robinson, C.A. (1988a) Reciprocal trust in health care relationships. *Journal of Advanced Nursing*, **13**(6), 782–9.

Thorne, S.E. & Robinson, C.A. (1988b) Health care relationships: the chronic illness perspective. *Research in Nursing and Health*, **11**(5), 293–300.

Thornes, R. (1983a) Parental access and family facilities in children's wards in England. *British Medical Journal*, **287**, 190–92.

Thornes, R. (1983b) *Parental Access and Overnight Accommodation in Children's Wards in England: The Regional Picture*. National Association for the Welfare of Children in Hospital, now Action for Sick Children, London.

Turner, J. (1984) A parent's perspective. *Nursing Mirror*, **159**(18), 23–5.

Webb, B. (1977) Trauma and tedium. In *Medical Encounters: the Experience of Illness and Treatment* (eds A. Davis & G. Horobin). Croom Helm, Beckenham, Kent.

Webb, N., Hull, D. & Madeley, R. (1985) Care by parents in hospital. *British Medical Journal*, **291**(6489), 176–7.

Wolfe, L. (1985) *Parental Access and Family Facilities in Wards Admitting Children in Scotland*. National Association for the Welfare of Children in Hospital, now Action for Sick Children, London.

Acknowledgements

The chapters in this book are updated papers originally published in the *Journal of Advanced Nursing*. Listed below are references to the original versions.

1 *The function of home visits in maternal and child welfare as evaluated by service providers and users* by Katri Vehviläinen-Julkunen: *Journal of Advanced Nursing* (1994) **20**, 672–8.
2 *Failure to immunize children under 5 years: a literature review* by Y.J. Lochhead: *Journal of Advanced Nursing* (1991) **16**, 130–37.
3 *Middle-Eastern immigrant parents' social networks and help-seeking for child health care* by Kathleen M.May: *Journal of Advanced Nursing* (1992) **17**, 905–12.
4 *School nursing* by Alison E. While and K. Louise Barriball: *Journal of Advanced Nursing* (1993) **18**, 1202–11.
5 *An assessment of the value of health education in the prevention of childhood asthma* by Doreen M. Deaves: *Journal of Advanced Nursing* (1993) **18**, 354–63.
6 *Familial inflammatory bowel disease in a paediatric population* by Gloria Joachim and Eric Hassall: *Journal of Advanced Nursing* (1992) **17**, 1310–16.
7 *Parents' experience of coming to know the care of a chronically ill child* by Mary D. Jerrett: *Journal of Advanced Nursing* (1994) **19**, 1050–56.
8 *Preparing children and families for day surgery* by Mary-Lou Ellerton and Craig Merriam: *Journal of Advanced Nursing* (1994) **19**, 1057–62.
9 *Analysed interaction in a children's oncology clinic: the child's view and parent's opinion of the effect of medical encounters* by Christine E. Inman: *Journal of Advanced Nursing* (1991) **16**, 782–93.
10 *Factors influencing nurses' pain assessment and interventions in children* by J.P.H. Hamers, H. Huijer Abu-Saad, R.J.G. Halfens and J.N.M. Schumacher: *Journal of Advanced Nursing* (1994) **20**, 853–60.
11 *The changing role of the nurse in neonatal care: a study of current practice in England* by Anne Harris and Margaret Redshaw: *Journal of Advanced Nursing* (1994) **20**, 874–80.
12 *Parents, nurses and paediatric nursing: a critical review* by Philip Darbyshire: *Journal of Advanced Nursing* (1993) **18**, 1670–80.

Index